T0221460

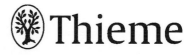

Passing the FRCR Part 1: Cracking Anatomy

Edited by

Niall Moore, MA (Cantab), MB BChir, FRCR, FRCP
Associate Professor of Radiology
Radiology Department
John Radcliffe Hospital
Oxford, United Kingdom

Authors

Yu-Yul Bashir, MB BS
Specialty Registrar, Oxford University Hospitals
Oxford, United Kingdom

Jane Chen, MB ChB, BSc, MRCP
Specialty Registrar, Oxford University Hospitals
Oxford, United Kingdom

Hassan Elhassan, BM BS
Specialty Registrar, Oxford University Hospitals
Oxford, United Kingdom

Jean Lee, MA (Cantab), MB BChir, MRCP
Specialty Registrar, Oxford University Hospitals
Oxford, United Kingdom

Heiko Peschl, BSc (Hons), MB BChir, MRCP
Specialty Registrar, Oxford University Hospitals
Oxford, United Kingdom

Matt Smedley, MB ChB, BSc
Specialty Registrar, Oxford University Hospitals
Oxford, United Kingdom

Thieme
Stuttgart • New York • Delhi • Rio

Library of Congress
Cataloging-in-Publication Data

Passing the FRCR Part 1: cracking anatomy / edited by Dr. Niall Moore, Dr. Yu-Yul Bashir, Dr. Jane Chen, Dr. Hassan Elhassan, Dr. Jean Lee, Dr. Heiko Peschl, Dr. Matt Smedley.

    p. ; cm.
    Cracking anatomy
    Includes index.
    ISBN 978-3-13-198761-7 – ISBN 978-3-13-198771-6 (eISBN)
I. Moore, Niall, editor of compilation. II. Title: Cracking anatomy.
[DNLM: 1. Anatomy–Great Britain–Examination Questions. 2. Radiology–Great Britain–Examination Questions. QS 18.2]
QM32
611.0076–dc23

                                  2013050895

©2014 Georg Thieme Verlag KG

Thieme Publishers Stuttgart
Rüdigerstrasse 14, 70469 Stuttgart, Germany
+49 [0]711 8931 421, customerservice@thieme.de

Thieme Publishers New York
333 Seventh Avenue, New York, NY 10001 USA
+1 800 782 3488, customerservice@thieme.com

Thieme Publishers Delhi
A-12, Second Floor, Sector-2, Noida-201301
Uttar Pradesh, India
+91 120 45 566 00, customerservice@thieme.in

Thieme Publishers Rio, Thieme Publicações Ltda.
Argentina Building 16th floor, Ala A, 228 Praia do Botafogo
Rio de Janeiro 22250-040 Brazil
+55 21 3736-3631

Cover design: Thieme Publishing Group
Typesetting by DiTech
Printed in Germany by Cuno GmbH

ISBN 978-3-13-198761-7

Also available as an e-book:
eISBN 978-3-13-198771-6

Important note: Medicine is an ever-changing science undergoing continual development. Research and clinical experience are continually expanding our knowledge, in particular our knowledge of proper treatment and drug therapy. Insofar as this book mentions any dosage or application, readers may rest assured that the authors, editors, and publishers have made every effort to ensure that such references are in accordance with the state of knowledge at the time of production of the book.

Nevertheless, this does not involve, imply, or express any guarantee or responsibility on the part of the publishers in respect to any dosage instructions and forms of applications stated in the book. Every user is requested to examine carefully the manufacturers' leaflets accompanying each drug and to check, if necessary in consultation with a physician or specialist, whether the dosage schedules mentioned therein or the contraindications stated by the manufacturers differ from the statements made in the present book. Such examination is particularly important with drugs that are either rarely used or have been newly released on the market. Every dosage schedule or every form of application used is entirely at the user's own risk and responsibility. The authors and publishers request every user to report to the publishers any discrepancies or inaccuracies noticed. If errors in this work are found after publication, errata will be posted at www.thieme.com on the product description page.

Some of the product names, patents, and registered designs referred to in this book are in fact registered trademarks or proprietary names even though specific reference to this fact is not always made in the text. Therefore, the appearance of a name without designation as proprietary is not to be construed as a representation by the publisher that it is in the public domain. This book, including all parts thereof, is legally protected by copyright. Any use, exploitation, or commercialization outside the narrow limits set by copyright legislation, without the publisher's consent, is illegal and liable to prosecution. This applies in particular to photostat reproduction, copying, mimeographing, preparation of microfilms, and electronic data processing and storage.

Contents

Preface

In Spring 2013, the format of the anatomy module of the Part 1 FRCR examination was changed. Previously, the examination consisted of 75 images, each with 5 questions relating to the normal anatomy being demonstrated. The questions typically asked the candidate to name the normal structures being pointed at. Now there are 100 images, each with 1 question corresponding to the image. As before, the candidate is typically asked to name a structure that has been labelled or to describe the normal variant demonstrated in the image.

Having taken the new examination whilst using revision material aimed at the old format, we realised that the approach to answering the questions is different and therefore an up-to-date revision aid to reflect this would be beneficial to the next cohort of candidates.

Handy hints for the examination

- The anatomy to be tested has been divided into four broad categories:
  - Head, neck, and spine
  - Chest and cardiovascular
  - Abdomen and pelvis
  - Musculoskeletal
- The examination consists of 25 questions on each of the four categories.
- There will also be an even spread of the modalities tested with a third of the questions devoted to the following:
  - Cross-sectional techniques (computed tomography [CT], magnetic resonance imaging [MRI], and ultrasound [US])
  - Plain radiographs
  - Contrast studies
- When only a single structure is labelled, as will be the case in the new style anatomy module, it can be easy to become fixated on the structure and to ignore the rest of the image. This is not a problem if you know the answer; however, if you are uncertain, you need to take note of the surrounding structures, which will help to orientate you to the position within the body and decide what the answer is.

- You will find that a number of questions use similar images. If you are struggling to identify the anatomy on one image and have seen a similar image elsewhere in the examination, you can try to use it to work out what the arrowed structure is. However, it is important not to spend too much time on one question. Instead, move on and return to it once you have completed the other questions.
- It can be difficult to know how much detail to provide for each answer. The advice from the Royal College of Radiologists (RCR) is to provide as much information as you would expect to see in a written radiology report. Always state whether the structure is left or right if it is a paired structure. Do not use abbreviations.
- Quite frequently, the question will relate to a structure that is shown on an unfamiliar plane. For example, we are all used to looking at the fourth ventricle in the sagittal plane; however, the examination may display it in the axial plane. The best way to deal with this during your revision is to make sure that you cover the main structures in all three planes in anatomy atlases. Whilst looking at cross sectional imaging at work, you should use a split screen and have all three planes displayed. If available, use a cross referencing tool to link the three planes together, scroll through the image, and try to familiarise yourself with the appearances of all the major anatomy in the three planes.

What to expect during the examination

- The RCR has now moved into the digital age with the introduction of the OsiriX© system into the Part 1 FRCR examination.
- The OsiriX© system is a Mac-only DICOM viewer that allows the user to view DICOM images and to make minor adjustments such as windowing the image.
- OsiriX© is available to MacOS X users for free. Simply type 'OsiriX' into your favourite search engine to find it.
- The examination is 90 minutes long and consists of 100 questions.

- The examination has two practice questions at the start, which will help to orientate you to the OsiriX© system.
- You will be seated at a computer station, which you will use to view the images. You will be provided with a pen, pencil, eraser, and pencil sharpener.
- You are not permitted to take anything into the examination, including your own writing equipment or water.
- There is one question per image. Make sure that you read the question carefully. Most often, the question is 'Name the arrowed structure'; however, occasionally, the question will differ, such as 'Name the structure that passes through this foramen'.

- You will be awarded two marks for a complete answer, one mark for a partially correct answer (for example, if you write the name of the structure but do not identify whether it is left or right), and zero marks if the answer is completely incorrect.
- There is no negative marking, so you should attempt to answer all questions.
- Finally, the College has provided a comprehensive section on its website covering all aspects of the examination, including a very useful FAQs section. Make sure that you visit the website prior to the examination to re-familiarise yourself and keep informed of any unexpected changes to the format.

Good luck!

Acknowledgments

Radiologists are clinical anatomists; anatomy is our stock-in-trade. A solid working knowledge of anatomy is essential, and it has always been tested searchingly by the Royal College of Radiologists. The examination is regularly reviewed, and the format has changed again. I am very grateful to the six authors of this revision book, who have specifically structured the text and chosen the images to prepare candidates for the new style of the Part 1 FRCR examination.

–Niall Moore, MA (Cantab), MB BChir, FRCR, FRCP

Chapter 1

Neuroanatomy and Head & Neck Anatomy

Question 1:

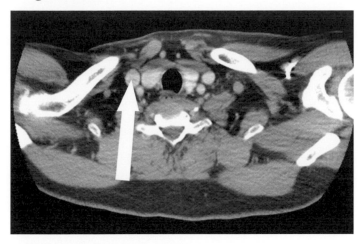

Name the arrowed structure	

Question 2:

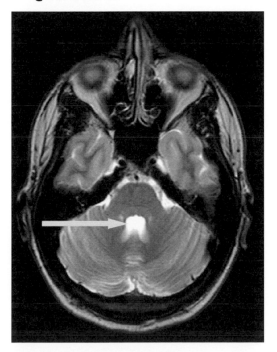

Name the arrowed structure	

■ Question 1: Axial CT of the neck

Answer: Right internal jugular vein

- The internal jugular vein is a continuation of the sigmoid sinus and is formed at the jugular foramen.
- It joins the subclavian vein to become the brachiocephalic vein posterior to the medial aspect of the clavicle.
- The internal jugular vein travels within the carotid sheath along with the common carotid artery. The vein is usually lateral to the artery and larger in diameter.
- It is usual for the left and right jugular veins to be of different calibre, often even more marked than in this case.

■ Question 2: Axial T2-weighted MRI of the brain

Answer: Fourth ventricle

- The fourth ventricle is a diamond-shaped structure that lies posterior to the pons.
- It is connected to the third ventricle superiorly via the aqueduct of Sylvius and to the central canal of the spinal cord inferiorly.
- It is also connected to the basal cisterns. One median aperture called the foramen of Magendie opens into the cisterna magna, whilst two lateral apertures called the foramina of Luschka open out into the cerebellopontine angle cisterns.

Question 3:

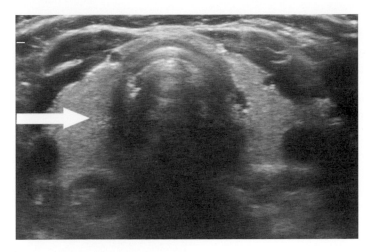

Name the arrowed structure	

Question 4:

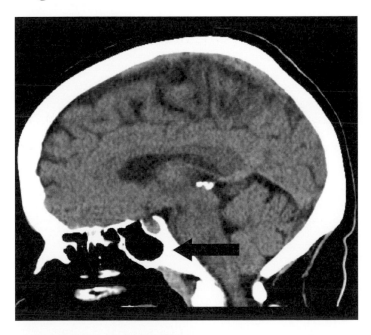

Name the arrowed structure	

■ Question 3: Ultrasound of the neck

Answer: Right lobe of thyroid gland

- On ultrasound, the thyroid gland can be recognised as a reflective, homogeneous structure with a grainy texture in the midline of the neck.
- The right lobe is often larger than the left.
- Each lobe is approximately 4 cm in height when imaged in the longitudinal plane.
- The trachea, seen between the two lobes of the gland, is a useful landmark.

■ Question 4: Sagittal CT of the brain

Answer: Clivus

- *Clivus* is Latin for 'slope'.
- It slopes obliquely in the midline.
- It lies posterior to the dorsum sellae and sphenoid sinus and anterior to the basilar artery and pons.
- It includes the posterior aspect of the body of the sphenoid bone and the basilar portion of the occipital bone.

Question 5:

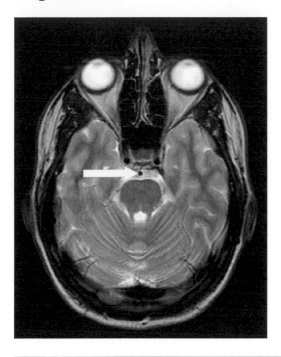

Name the arrowed structure	

■ Question 5: Axial T2-weighted MRI of the brain

Answer: Basilar artery

- The basilar artery is a single vessel in the midline and is part of the posterior circulation.
- It lies posterior to the dorsum sellae and clivus and anterior to the pons.
- It arises from the paired vertebral arteries at the base of the pons.
- It gives off the following paired branches:
  - Anterior inferior cerebellar artery
  - Labyrinthine artery (variable)
  - Pontine artery
  - Superior cerebellar artery
- The basilar artery terminates at the paired posterior cerebral arteries.

■ Question 6:

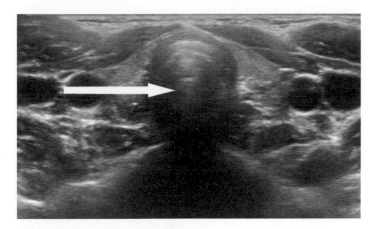

Name the arrowed structure	

■ Question 7:

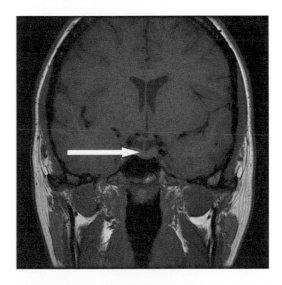

Name the arrowed structure	

■ Question 6: Ultrasound of the neck

Answer: Trachea

- The trachea lies in the midline between the two lobes of the thyroid gland.
- Anteriorly, a tracheal ring can be seen. Fifteen to twenty incomplete cartilaginous rings make up the trachea.
- Posteriorly, an acoustic shadow is formed by the air within the trachea, which is a poor ultrasound medium and prevents visualisation of deeper structures.

■ Question 7: Coronal T1-weighted MRI of the brain

Answer: Pituitary gland

- The pituitary gland is harder to recognise on coronal images given that you will be more used to looking at it on sagittal views.
- There are several clues that will help you identify this structure.
  - It sits within a depression in the sphenoid sinus—this is the sella turcica.
  - There is a stalk arising from its superior aspect—this is the infundibulum.
  - It is a midline structure.
  - The optic chiasm is superior.

Question 8:

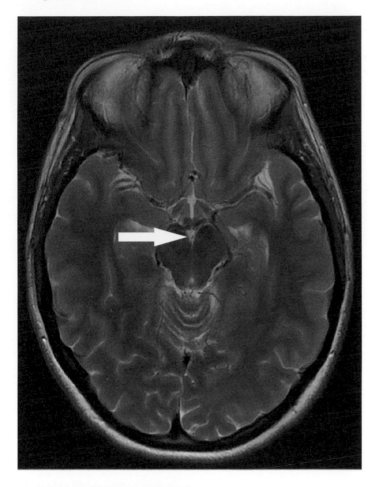

Name the arrowed structure	

■ Question 8: Axial T2-weighted MRI of the brain

Answer: Interpeduncular cistern

- This portion of the brainstem is the midbrain, which somewhat resembles the head of Mickey Mouse.
- Between the cerebral peduncles (which are the ears of Mickey Mouse) lies the interpeduncular fossa. The interpeduncular cistern is located within the interpeduncular fossa.
- It lies posterior to the optic chiasm.

■ Question 9:

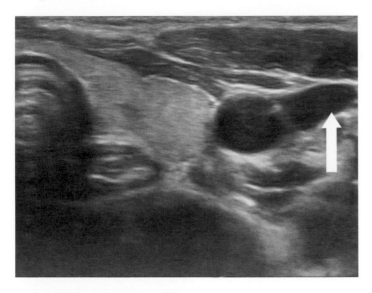

Name the arrowed structure	

■ Question 10:

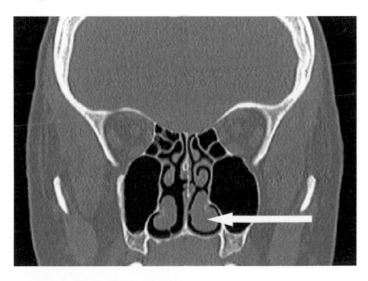

Name the arrowed structure	

■ Question 9: Ultrasound of the neck

Answer: Left internal jugular vein

- On ultrasound, blood vessels are anechoic structures.
- The internal jugular vein is usually lateral and slightly posterior to the common carotid artery. It is normally of a larger calibre compared to the artery but, in this case, the vein is not fully distended.

■ Question 10: Coronal CT of the brain

Answer: Left inferior nasal turbinate bone

- The turbinates are respiratory epithelium-lined, curled bones in the lateral portion of the nasal cavity.
- They are divided by the nasal septum in the midline.
- There are three pairs of nasal turbinates:
  - Inferior turbinates (the largest)
  - Middle turbinates
  - Superior turbinates

■ Question 11:

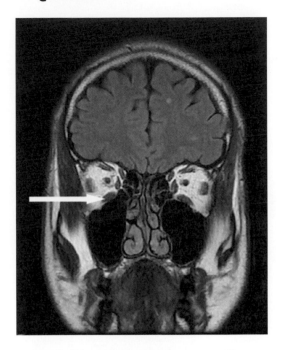

Name the arrowed structure	

■ Question 11: Coronal MRI of the brain

Answer: Right inferior rectus muscle

- The inferior rectus muscle is a paired structure that depresses the eye.
- It is innervated by the oculomotor nerve.
- It is one of the six extraocular muscles of the orbit. See figure below.

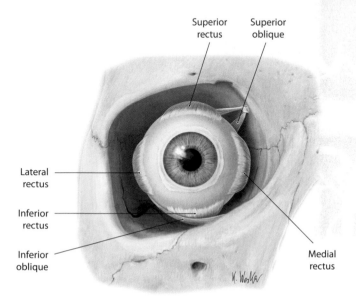

From Atlas of Anatomy, © Thieme 2008, illustration by Karl Wesker.

▪ Question 12:

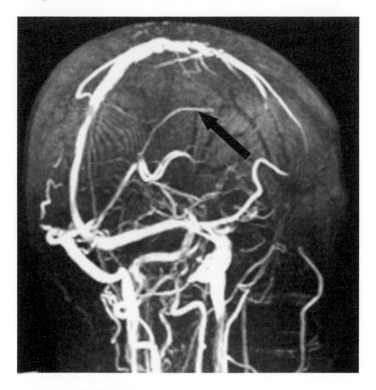

Name the arrowed structure	

■ Question 12: MR venogram

Answer: Inferior sagittal sinus

- The inferior sagittal sinus runs along the inferior border of the falx cerebri.
- It drains into the straight sinus, as does the great cerebral vein of Galen.
- It can be distinguished from the great vein by the fact that it parallels the course of the superior sagittal sinus.
- The figure below shows the main dural venous sinuses.

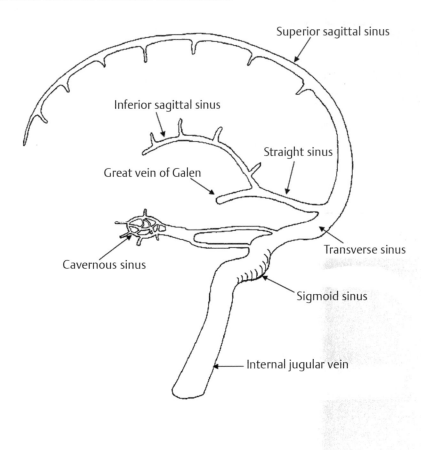

■ Question 13:

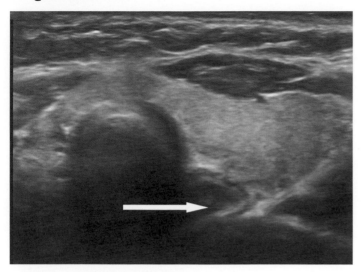

Name the arrowed structure	

■ Question 14:

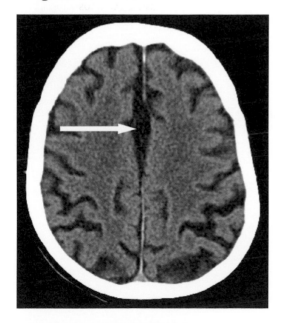

Name the arrowed structure	

■ Question 13: Ultrasound of the neck

Answer: Oesophagus

- The oesophagus lies to the left of the trachea, posterior to the left lobe of the thyroid.
- There are specks of increased reflectivity within the lumen that are caused by the presence of air within the oesophagus.
- You can also see the layers of muscle in the wall of the oesophagus.

■ Question 14: Axial CT of the brain

Answer: Interhemispheric fissure

- An interhemispheric fissure is a deep groove running from anterior to posterior in the midline that separates the left and right cerebral hemispheres.
- The falx cerebri runs through the fissure as shown in the image.

Question 15:

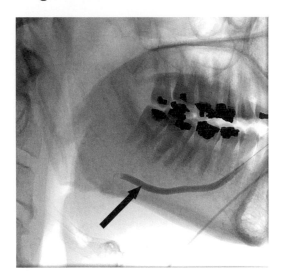

Name the arrowed structure	

Question 16:

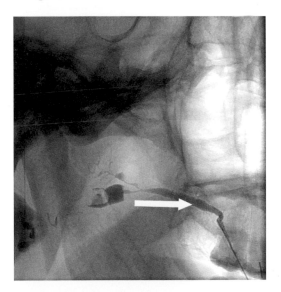

Name the arrowed structure	

▪ Question 15: Sialogram

Answer: Submandibular (Wharton's) duct

- The submandibular duct drains saliva produced by the submandibular gland into the floor of the mouth at the base of the tongue.
- The duct is approximately 5 cm long.

▪ Question 16: Sialogram

Answer: Parotid (Stensen's) duct

- The parotid duct conveys saliva from the parotid gland into the oral cavity.
- The gland opens out into the mucosal surface of the inner cheek opposite the upper second molar tooth.
- Initially, it is difficult to ascertain what the image shows. Images like this can appear in the examination and the best way to tackle a confusing one is to find recognisable landmarks. If you look carefully, you will see that the mandibular condyle can be discerned on the left side of the image, and teeth can be seen at the bottom right-hand corner.
- By finding these landmarks, you will be guided as to which body part is being shown.

■ Question 17:

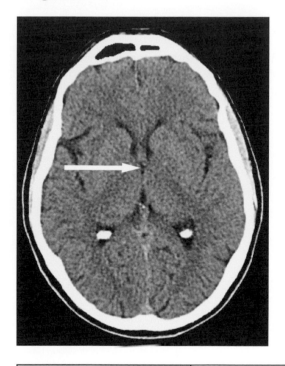

Name the arrowed structure	

■ Question 17: Axial CT of the brain

Answer: Third ventricle

- The third ventricle is a slitlike structure in the midline that is filled with cerebrospinal fluid.
- It is connected to the lateral ventricles by the foramina of Monro and to the fourth ventricle by the aqueduct of Sylvius.
- The thalami sit on either side of the third ventricle.

Question 18:

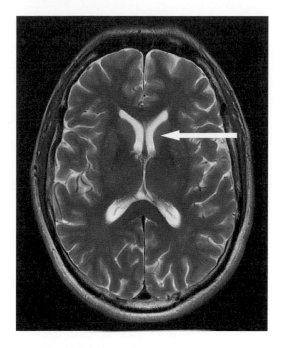

Name the arrowed structure	

■ Question 18: Axial T2-weighted MRI of the brain

Answer: Head of the left caudate nucleus

- The caudate nucleus lies lateral to the frontal horn of the lateral ventricle and medial to the internal capsule.
- The caudate consists of the head, body, and tail (posterior).
- Putamen + caudate nucleus = striatum

Question 19:

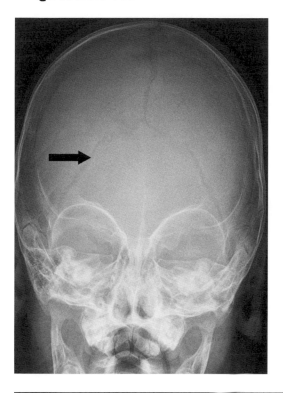

Name the arrowed structure	

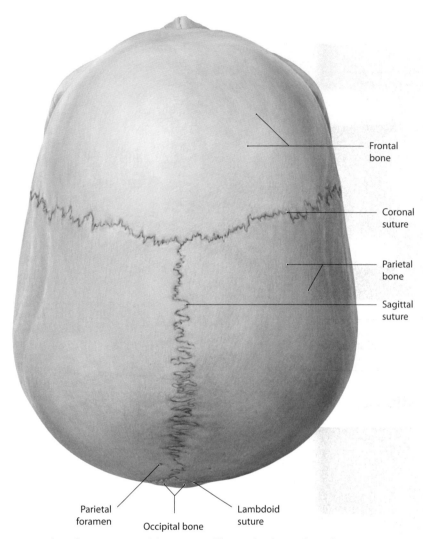

Frontal
bone

Coronal
suture

Parietal
bone

Sagittal
suture

Parietal
foramen

Occipital bone

Lambdoid
suture

From Atlas of Anatomy, © Thieme 2008, illustration by Karl Wesker.

▪ Question 20:

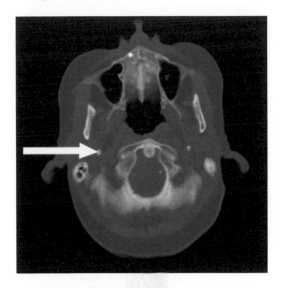

Name the arrowed structure	

▪ Question 21:

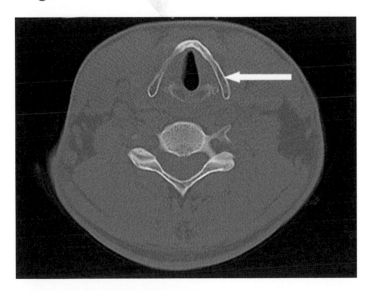

Name the arrowed structure	

■ Question 20: Axial CT of the skull base

Answer: Right styloid process

- The styloid process is a long and slender projection of the petrous temporal bone.
- It is the site of attachment of three muscles: the styloglossus, stylohyoid, and stylopharyngeus.
- On axial imaging, the styloid process appears as a small, rounded segment of bone between the ramus of the mandible anteriorly and the mastoid air cells posteriorly.

■ Question 21: Axial CT of the neck

Answer: Thyroid cartilage

- When viewed anteriorly, the thyroid cartilage is a shield-shaped structure that is composed of two flat plates (laminae) that converge in the midline to form the laryngeal prominence.
- The epiglottis is attached to the inner surface of the thyroid cartilage at the midline.
- Extending from the posterior border of each lamina are superior and inferior horns to which numerous muscles of the larynx attach.

■ Question 22:

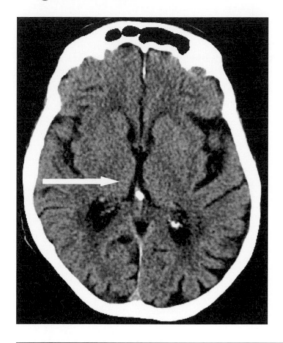

Name the arrowed structure	

■ Question 22: Axial CT of the brain

Answer: Right thalamus

- The thalamus is a paired, walnut-shaped, deep grey matter multinuclear structure that lies on either side of the third ventricle and anterior to the occipital horn of the lateral ventricles.
- It acts as a sensory and motor synaptic relay centre.

Question 23:

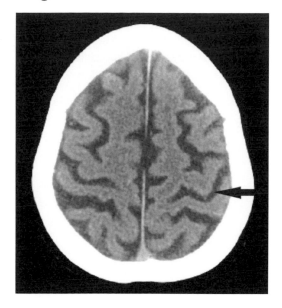

Name the arrowed structure	

Question 24:

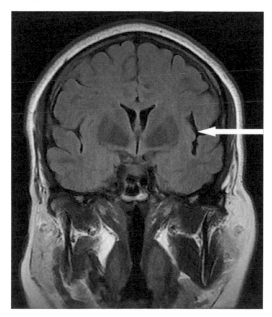

Name the arrowed structure	

▪ Question 25: MR venogram (MIP image)

Answer: Superior sagittal sinus

- The superior sagittal sinus is part of the venous drainage system of the brain.
- The superior sagittal sinus travels from anteriorly to posteriorly within the falx cerebri.
- It is a midline structure that drains into the confluence of the sinuses (torcular herophili) at the internal occipital protuberance.
- It receives blood from both the superficial cerebral veins and the deep cerebral veins.

▪ Question 26:

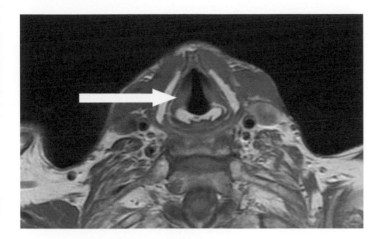

Name the arrowed structure	

▪ Question 27:

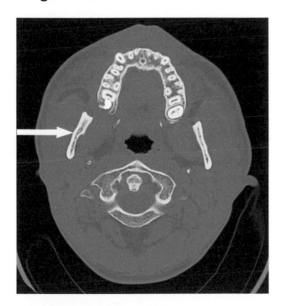

Name the arrowed structure	

▪ Question 26: Axial T1-weighted MRI of the neck

Answer: Right vocal cord

- The true vocal cords are part of the glottis—the portion of the larynx that is triangular in cross section.
- The mucosa of the larynx wraps around the vocal ligaments to form the true cords, which are responsible for phonation.
- Superior to this, the laryngeal mucosa folds around the vestibular ligaments to form the false cords.

▪ Question 27: Axial CT of the head

Answer: Right ramus of the mandible

- The ramus of the mandible is the posterior vertical extension of the body of the mandible.
- The superior mandibular ramus divides into the coronoid process (anteriorly) and the condyloid process extending to the mandibular condyle (posteriorly).

■ Question 28:

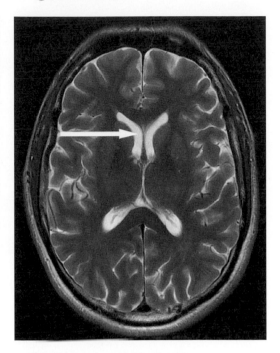

Name the arrowed structure	

■ Question 29:

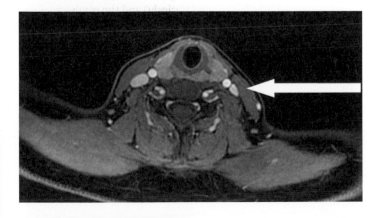

Name the arrowed structure	

■ Question 28: Axial T2-weighted MRI of the brain

Answer: Frontal horn of the right lateral ventricle

- The lateral ventricles are paired C-shaped structures.
- They consist of the frontal horn, body (central part), temporal (inferior) horn, and the occipital (posterior) horn.
- They contain the choroid plexus, which produces the cerebrospinal fluid.

■ Question 29: Axial T2-weighted MRI of the neck

Answer: Left sternocleidomastoid muscle

- The sternocleidomastoid muscle lies anterolateral to the carotid sheath and is the largest muscle in the anterior part of the neck.
- The sternocleidomastoid muscle divides the neck into an anterior triangle and a posterior triangle. It is an important landmark when describing lymph node levels in the neck.

Question 30:

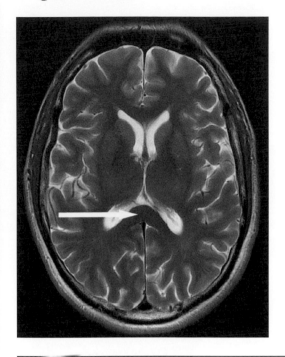

Name the arrowed structure	

▪ Question 30: Axial T2-weighted MRI of the brain

Answer: Splenium of corpus callosum

- This is a midline structure that crosses the interhemispheric fissure and facilitates communication between the left and right cerebral hemispheres.

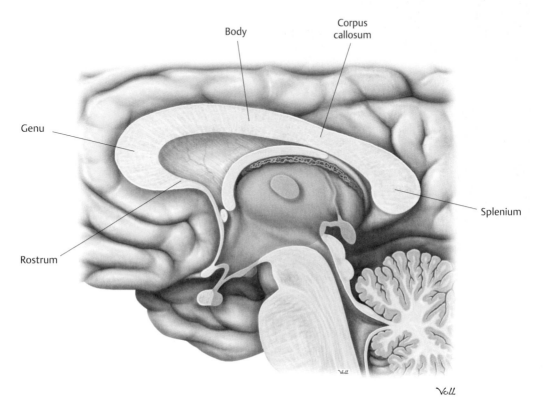

From Atlas of Anatomy, © Thieme 2008, illustration by Markus Voll.

Question 31:

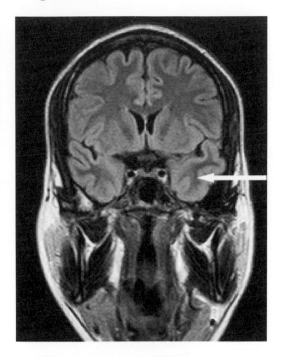

Name the arrowed structure	

■ Question 31: Coronal MRI of the brain

Answer: Left temporal lobe (white matter)

- The temporal lobes are the most inferior lobes of the cerebral cortex.
- The temporal lobes occupy the middle cranial fossae.
- They are separated from the superior frontal lobes by the Sylvian (lateral) fissures (pictured).
- They contain the limbic system.

Question 32:

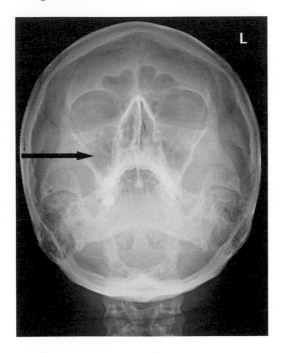

Name the arrowed structure	

▪ Question 32: Radiograph of the face (occipitomental 30° projection)

Answer: Right maxillary sinus

- The maxillary sinus, or antrum, is a pyramidal mucosa-lined air space in the body of the maxilla.
- It is inferior to the orbits and lateral to the nasal cavity.
- It is the largest of the paranasal sinuses.
- It drains into the middle meatus of the nose.

Question 33:

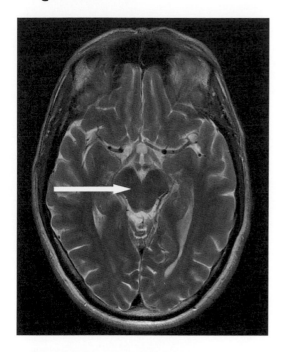

Name the arrowed structure	

Question 34:

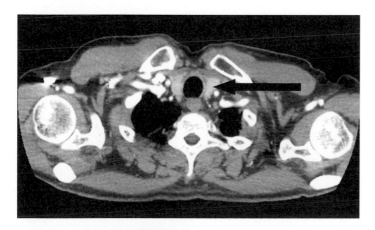

Name the arrowed structure	

▪ Question 33: Axial T2-weighted MRI brain

Answer: Midbrain

- The midbrain is the most superior portion of the brainstem.
- On axial images, it is 'Mickey Mouse'–shaped; the cerebral peduncles resemble the ears.
- It connects to the thalamus (superiorly) and to the pons (inferiorly).
- The midbrain is divided into three portions:
  - Tectum (posterior)
    - Made up of the tectal/quadrigeminal plate and the superior and inferior colliculi
  - Tegmentum
  - Cerebral peduncles (anterior)
    - Separated by the interpeduncular fossa in the midline, which contains the mamillary bodies

▪ Question 34: Axial CT at the level of the lung apices

Answer: Left lobe of the thyroid gland

- On CT, the thyroid gland can be recognised as a midline structure on either side of the trachea; the thyroid has a higher attenuation than the rest of the soft tissues due to its high iodine content.

Question 35:

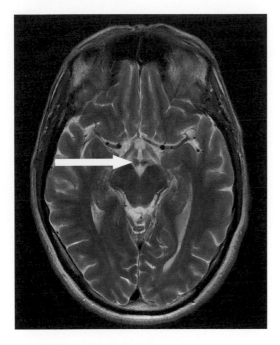

Name the arrowed structure	

■ Question 35: Axial T2-weighted MRI of the brain

Answer: Right mamillary body

- The mamillary body is a paired, small, round structure located in the interpeduncular cistern/fossa.
- It extends from the hypothalamus.
- It returns low signal on a T2-weighted MRI.

■ Question 36:

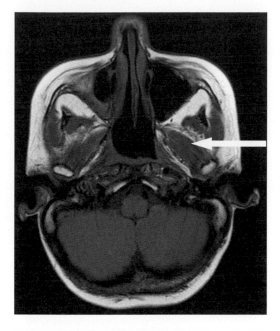

Name the arrowed structure	

■ Question 36: T1-weighted MRI of the skull base

Answer: Left lateral pterygoid muscle

- The lateral pterygoid is a muscle of mastication with two heads.
- The upper head arises from the greater wing of the sphenoid bone and inserts onto the articular disc of the temporomandibular joint.
- The lower head arises from the lateral pterygoid plate and inserts onto the neck of the mandibular condyle as demonstrated on the image.

- **Question 37:**

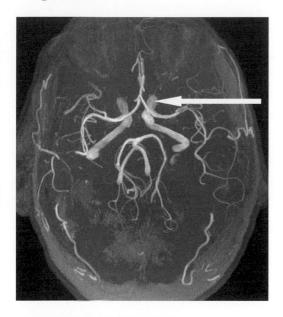

Name the arrowed structure	

▪ Question 37: MR angiogram of the circle of Willis (MIP image)

Answer: Left internal carotid artery

- The internal carotid arteries arise from the bifurcation of the common carotid arteries at the level of C4 and ascend to the base of the skull.
- They then enter the cranial cavity via the carotid canal in the petrous bone and follow a tortuous course before terminating at the anterior perforated substance by dividing into the anterior and middle cerebral arteries.
- At the circle of Willis, the internal carotid arteries can be recognised as the vessels with the greatest diameters.

■ Question 38:

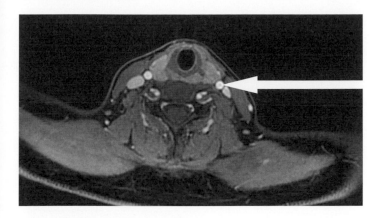

Name the arrowed structure	

■ Question 39:

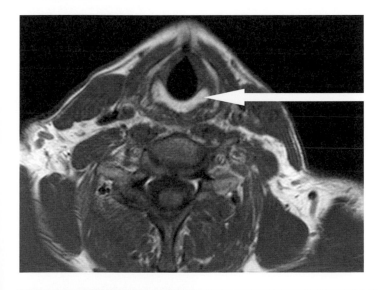

Name the arrowed structure	

▪ Question 38: T1-weighted, fat-suppressed, contrast-enhanced MRI of the neck

Answer: Left common carotid artery

- The left common carotid artery arises from the arch of the aorta and ascends into the neck.
- It travels in the carotid sheath with the internal jugular vein laterally and the vagus nerve posteriorly.
- The common carotid artery divides into the internal and external carotid arteries at the level of C4.

▪ Question 39: MRI of the neck

Answer: Cricoid cartilage

- The cricoid cartilage is part of the cartilaginous framework that surrounds the larynx.
- The cricoid cartilage lies inferior to the thyroid cartilage and articulates with its inferior horns as demonstrated on the image.
- Although not apparent on this CT image, the cricoid cartilage is actually a ringed structure. The posterior part of the ring is greater in length in the craniocaudal dimension than the anterior part; hence, the anterior part of the cartilage cannot be seen on the image.

Question 40:

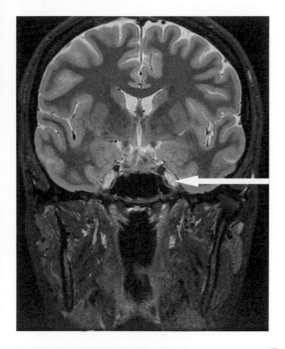

Name the arrowed structure	

▪ Question 40: Coronal T2-weighted MRI of the brain

Answer: Left Meckel's cave (trigeminal cave)

- Meckel's cave is a pouch containing cerebrospinal fluid formed by two layers of dura mater derived from the tentorium cerebelli.
- It contains the trigeminal nerve roots and ganglion.
- It lies adjacent to the posterolateral aspect of the cavernous sinus and lateral to the sphenoid bones.
- It is lateral to the internal carotid arteries.

Question 41:

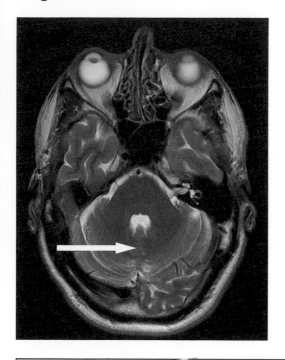

Name the arrowed structure	

■ Question 41: Axial T2-weighted MRI of the brain

Answer: Cerebellar vermis

- The cerebellar vermis is a single midline structure in the posterior fossa that connects the two cerebellar hemispheres.
- It lies posterior to the fourth ventricle.
- The vermis is separated into nine lobules by fissures (folia).

Question 42:

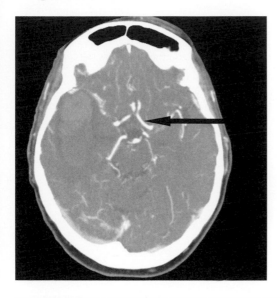

Name the arrowed structure	

■ Question 42: CT angiogram of the circle of Willis

Answer: Left anterior cerebral artery (ACA)

- The circle of Willis is more pentagonal in shape than circular.
- It encloses the optic chiasm and pituitary stalk.
- The left and right ACA form the roof of the pentagon and are joined together by the anterior communicating artery (which cannot be clearly visualised on the image).
- This is not the best example of the circle of Willis, but it has been included because the examples in the examination are sometimes purposefully not of the best quality to test your knowledge.
- The figure below shows all the branches that form the circle of Willis.

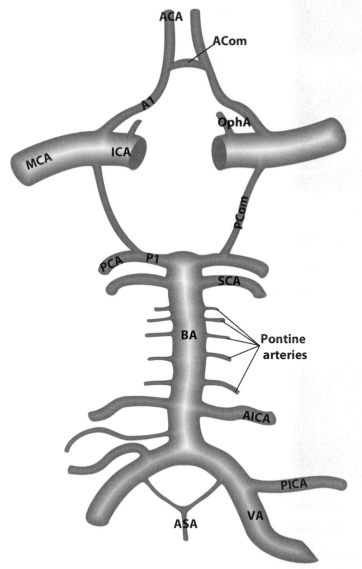

From Sanna M, Piazza P Shin S, et al. Microsurgery of Skull Base Paragangliomas. Stuttgart, Germany: Thieme Medical Publishers; 2013.

Question 43:

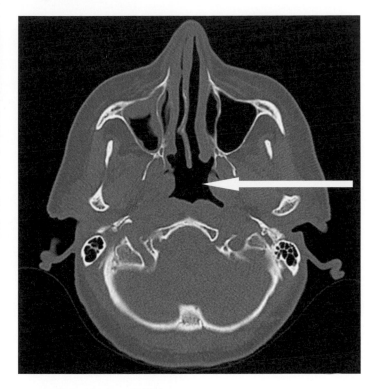

Name the arrowed structure	

Question 44:

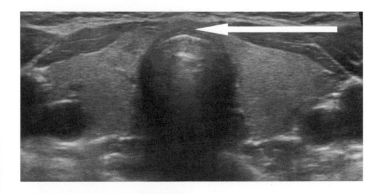

Name the arrowed structure	

■ Question 43: Axial CT of the skull

Answer: Nasopharynx

- The pharynx is a muscular tube that is part of both the respiratory and gastrointestinal tracts.
- It is divided into three parts: the nasopharynx, oropharynx, and hypopharynx.
- On an axial image, the nasopharynx can be identified by its anterior communication with the nasal cavity.

Question 44: Ultrasound of the neck

Answer: Isthmus

- The isthmus connects the two lobes of the thyroid gland and passes anterior to the trachea in the midline of the neck.
- A pyramidal lobe may extend cranially from the isthmus—this is a remnant of the thyroglossal duct.

Question 45:

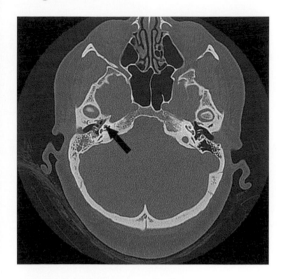

Name the arrowed structure	

▪ Question 45: Axial CT of the brain

Answer: Right cochlea

- The cochlea is a paired, spiral-shaped conical chamber that forms part of the vestibular system.
- *Cochlea* is Latin for 'snail shell'.
- It is part of the temporal bone and sits medial to the mastoid air cells and anterior to the vestibular aqueduct.

Question 46:

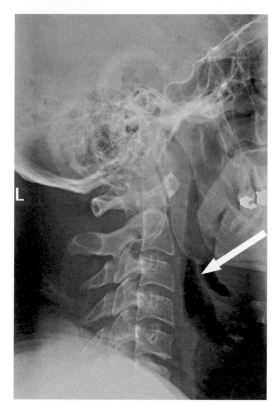

Name the arrowed structure	

■ Question 46: Lateral radiograph of the cervical spine

Answer: Epiglottis

- The epiglottis is a leaf-shaped cartilage.
- On a lateral radiograph, it can be recognised as a structure of soft tissue density arising from the laryngeal part of the pharynx, extending cranially into the oropharynx, posterior to the base of the tongue.
- During swallowing, it directs food boluses into the pyriform sinuses to protect the larynx.

Question 47:

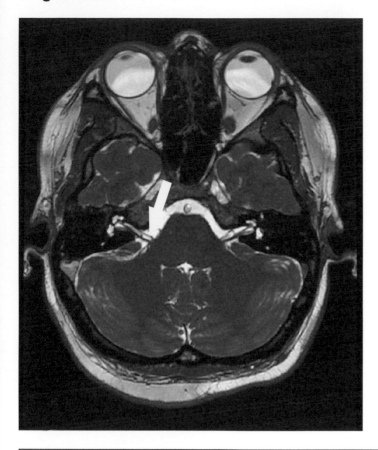

Name the arrowed structure	

▪ Question 47: Axial thin section T2-weighted MRI of the brain

Answer: Right facial nerve (CN VII)

- The facial nerve lies anterior to the vestibulocochlear nerve, which is also shown here.
- Moving more caudally, there are another two pairs of cranial nerves (CNs) that look very similar. They are the glossopharyngeal and vagus nerves.
- The best way to identify which pair is being shown is to look at the level of the brainstem and surrounding anatomy.
- CNs VII and VIII arise from the pons, as shown in the image. Note the other structures such as the orbits and temporal lobes. CNs IX and X are seen at the level of the medulla.

■ Question 48:

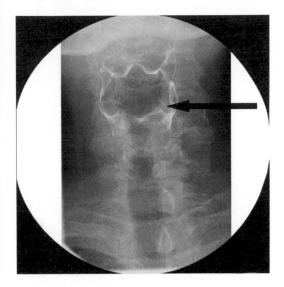

Name the arrowed structure	

▪ Question 48: Barium swallow

Answer: Left pyriform sinus

- The pyriform sinuses are a pair of deep recesses that lie on either side of the laryngeal orifice.
- They are bounded laterally by the thyroid cartilage.
- The valleculae can be seen superior to the pyriform sinuses.

Question 49:

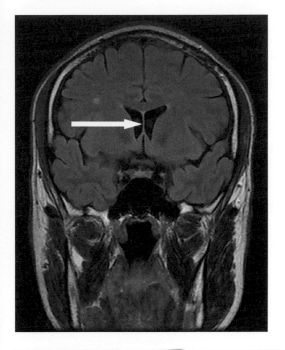

Name the arrowed structure	

■ Question 49: Coronal MRI of the brain

Answer: Septum pellucidum

- The septum pellucidum is a thin, vertical membrane in the midline extending from the corpus callosum to the fornix posteriorly.
- It separates the frontal horns of the left and right lateral ventricles.
- The septum pellucidum is situated anterior to the foramina of Monro.
- Normal variants:
  - Cavum septum pellucidum (anterior) and/or cavum septum vergae (posterior): Nonobliteration of the potential space between the leaflets of the septum pellucidum
  - Cavum velum interpositum: Dilated CSF-filled space involving the velum interpositum, which extends from the foramina of Monro to the quadrigeminal cistern

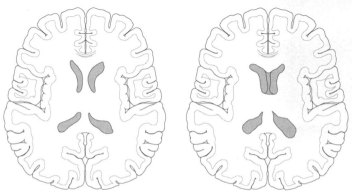

Normal   Cavum septum pellucidum

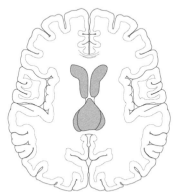

Cavum velum interpositum

▪ Question 50:

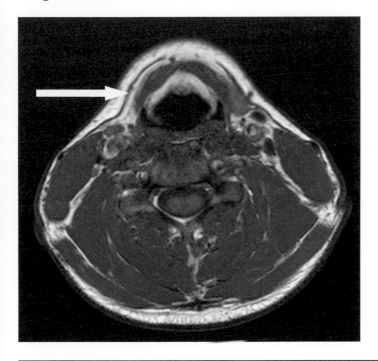

Name the arrowed structure	

■ Question 50: Axial T1-weighted MRI of the neck

Answer: Right platysma muscle

- The platysma is a broad but thin sheet of muscle that is derived from the fascia of the pectoralis major muscle and the deltoid muscle.
- It inserts onto the body of the mandible and onto the skin of the lower face.
- In humans, it is a muscle of facial expression; in horses, it is more developed and its contractions act to repel insects.
- It is the most superficial muscle in the anterior portion of the neck.
- The name is derived from the Greek word *platus*, which means wide.

Chapter 2

Chest and Cardiovascular Anatomy

Question 1:

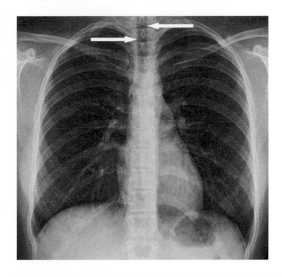

Name the arrowed structure	

Question 2:

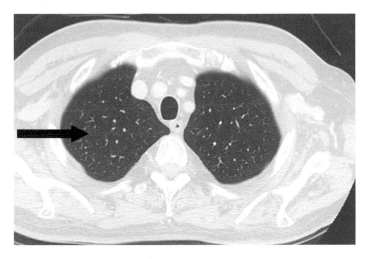

Name the arrowed structure	

▪ Question 1: PA chest radiograph

Answer: Trachea

- The trachea is a rigid, tubular structure responsible for the passage of air from the pharynx to the lungs and is reinforced by C-shaped cartilaginous rings. The flat band of muscle and connective tissue posterior to it is called the posterior tracheal membrane, which can appear convex during expiratory views on CT.
- It is 12 to 15 cm long in adults.
- On a PA chest radiograph, it is seen as a midline transradiant cylindrical structure beginning at the level of the lower part of the cricoid cartilage and extending to the carina (from C6 to approximately T5).
- A slight deviation to the right is normal, particularly in children.

▪ Question 2: Axial CT of the chest

Answer: Right upper lobe

- The right upper lobe is separated from the middle lobe by the horizontal fissure.
- It is divided into three segments: anterior, apical, and posterior.
- The interface between the right upper lobe medial pleural surface and right lateral tracheal border, when seen on a chest radiograph, is termed right paratracheal stripe.

Question 3:

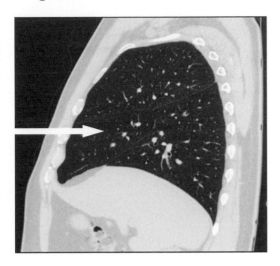

Name the arrowed structure	

Question 4:

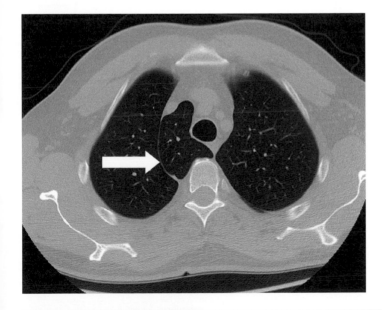

Name the arrowed structure	

▪ Question 3: Sagittal CT of the chest

Answer: Middle lobe

- The middle lobe is divided into two segments: medial and lateral.
- It is separated from the upper lobe by the horizontal fissure superiorly and from the lower lobe by the oblique fissure inferiorly.

▪ Question 4: Axial CT of the chest

Answer: Azygos fissure

- An azygos fissure is the most common accessory fissure and is a common examination question.
- An azygos fissure is seen in approximately 1% of the population.
- It occurs because of failure of normal migration of the azygos vein, which leads to invagination of the parietal and visceral pleura along its course. Sometimes the section of lung medial to the fissure is termed the azygos lobe.
- If complete, it has clinical relevance because it acts as a barrier to apical consolidation extending inferiorly to the rest of the upper lobe.

■ Question 5:

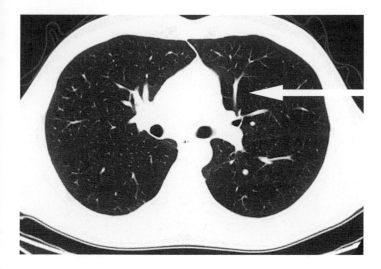

Name the arrowed structure	

■ Question 5: Axial CT of the chest

Answer: Left upper lobe

- The left upper lobe is analogous to a combined right upper and middle lobe.
- It is separated from the left lower lobe by the left oblique fissure.
- It is divided into four segments: anterior, apicoposterior, and the superior and inferior lingular segments.
- The figure below illustrates the different lung segments within the lung lobes with which you should familiarise yourself.

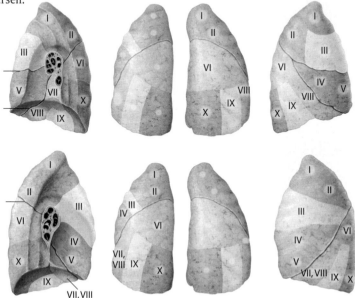

From Atlas of Anatomy, © Thieme 2008, illustrations by Markus Voll.

Segmental architecture of the lungs				
Each segment is supplied by a segmental bronchus of the same name (e.g., the apical segmental bronchus supplies the apical segment).				
Right lung		**Left lung**		
Superior lobe				
I	Apical segment	Apicoposterior segment		I
II	Posterior segment			II
III	Anterior segment			III
Middle lobe		**Lingula**		
IV	Lateral segment	Superior lingular segment		IV
V	Medial segment	Inferior lingular segment		V
Inferior lobe				
VI	Superior segment			VI
VII	Medial basal segment			VII
VIII	Anterior basal segment			VIII
IX	Lateral basal segment			IX
X	Posterior basal segment			X

Note: In the left lower lobe, the anterior basal and medial basal segments are conjoined to form the anteromedial basal segment.

Question 6:

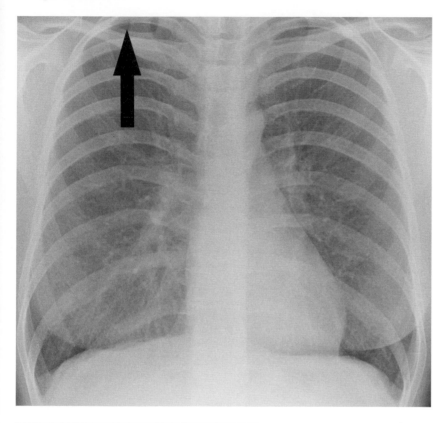

Name the arrowed structure	

▪ Question 6: PA chest radiograph

Answer: Companion shadow beside the right clavicle

- The companion shadow is the skin and subcutaneous fat that are seen as a thin soft tissue stripe along the upper edge of the clavicle. It should not be mistaken for an abnormality.
- Similar companion shadows can be formed by the ribs and scapulae. They are not always seen on a radiograph.

Question 7:

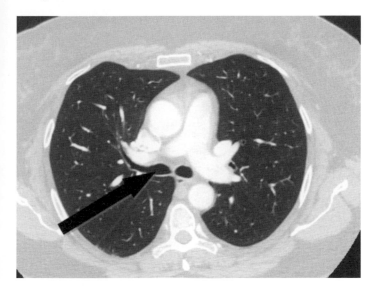

Name the arrowed structure	

Question 8:

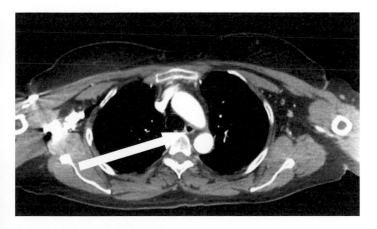

Name the arrowed structure	

■ Question 7: Axial CT of the chest

Answer: Right main bronchus

- The right main bronchus arises from the trachea at the carina.
- It forms a more obtuse angle with the trachea compared to the left (lies at 25° to the median plane).
- It is considerably shorter than the left (about half the length) with a mean length of 2.2 cm.

■ Question 8: Axial CT of the chest

Answer: Oesophagus

- The oesophagus is the muscular tubular structure that is responsible for conducting food from the mouth to the stomach. It begins at the level of the cricopharyngeus and terminates at the gastro-oesophageal junction and measures approximately 25 cm in length.
- The examination aims to test the candidate on common anatomical structures, but in somewhat unusual modalities or planes such as an axial CT in this instance, or a sagittal CT demonstrating a longitudinal 'slip' of air posterior to the trachea that may project in and out of plane.

Question 9:

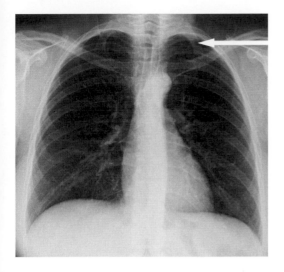

Name the arrowed structure	

■ Question 9: PA chest radiograph

Answer: Left first rib

- The first rib is the flattest and most curved rib.
- The first rib arises from the upward sloping transverse process of the first thoracic vertebra; this distinguishes it from a cervical rib, which arises from the downward sloping transverse process of the seventh cervical vertebra.

Question 10:

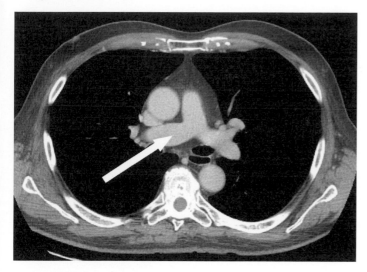

Name the arrowed structure	

Question 11:

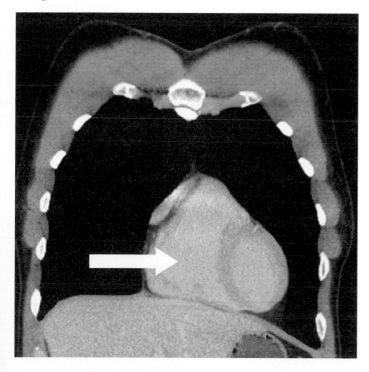

Name the arrowed structure	

▪ Question 10: Axial CT of the chest

Answer: Right main pulmonary artery

- The right main pulmonary artery arises at a right angle from the pulmonary trunk and passes behind the ascending aorta and the superior vena cava. It passes anterior to the right main bronchus.
- It is longer than the left main pulmonary artery.
- The left main pulmonary artery arches superiorly over the left bronchus making it much shorter. This is why the left hilar point is higher than the right on a PA chest radiograph.

▪ Question 11: Coronal CT of the chest

Answer: Right ventricle

- The right ventricle is an anterior structure and, when anatomically normal, is not visible on a PA radiograph. It is border-forming on a lateral projection.
- Being the second largest chamber in a normal heart, it is readily identifiable.
- Sometimes the right ventricle will be shown in alternative projections, such as sagittal views where its inferior border usually comes into contact with the sternum, or a coronal view (as in this case) to show its anterior position.

Question 12:

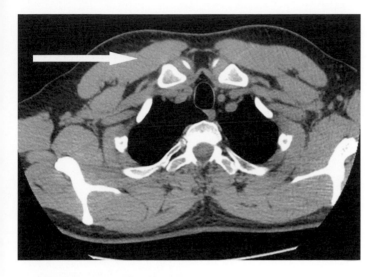

Name the arrowed structure	

Question 13:

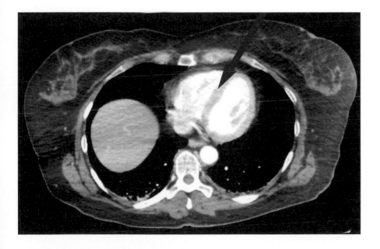

Name the arrowed structure	

■ Question 12: Axial CT of the chest

Answer: Right pectoralis major muscle

- The pectoralis major muscle is a fan-shaped muscle that covers the anterior superior aspect of the thorax and is the most superficial muscle.
- It has two components that are capable of acting independently: a sternal component and a clavicular component. These converge to cross below the shoulder joint to insert at the bicipital groove.
- The pectoralis major muscle is a strong adductor of the arm and also acts as an internal rotator of the humerus.

■ Question 13: Axial CT of the chest

Answer: Interventricular septum

- The interventricular septum is a strong, thick structure composed of muscular and membranous components that separate the ventricles. It bows to the right due to the higher left ventricular pressure.
- Assessment of the interventricular septum is important because it is a marker of many cardiopulmonary diseases such as pulmonary hypertension, ventricular septal defects, and interventricular aneurysms.

Question 14:

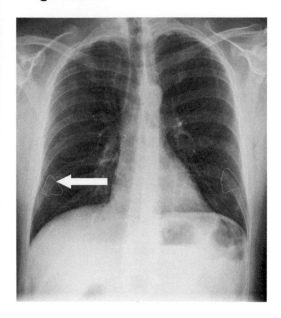

Name the arrowed structure	

▪ Question 14: PA chest radiograph

Answer: Right nipple marker

- A nipple marker is a high-density object (usually a metallic triangle or marker) that is placed over the nipple to help differentiate nipple shadows that appear as soft tissue densities from a true parenchymal nodule in erect chest radiographs.
- Nipple shadows, if present, have a characteristic location at the level of the fifth or the sixth anterior rib and often have a well-defined lateral margin; their location can vary with breast size.

Question 15:

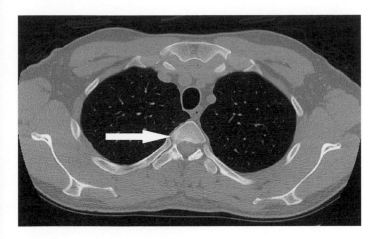

Name the arrowed structure	

Question 16:

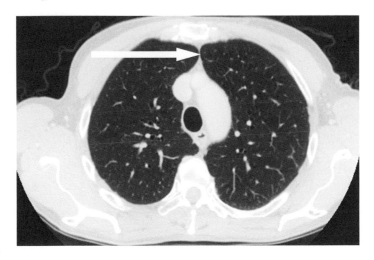

Name the arrowed structure	

▪ Question 15: Axial CT of the chest

Answer: Right costovertebral joint

- A costovertebral joint, as the name implies, is the articulation between the head of a rib and the vertebral column.
- A typical rib articulates at two points with the spine: the head of the rib articulates with the vertebral body (costovertebral) and the tubercle of the rib articulates with the transverse process (costotransverse).
- Atypical ribs such as the 11th and 12th ribs do not articulate with the corresponding transverse processes of the vertebral body.
- The costovertebral joint is a synovial joint and, as such, is prone to synovial disease processes such as rheumatoid arthritis.

▪ Question 16: Axial CT of the chest

Answer: Anterior junctional line

- The anterior junctional line is formed by the visceral and parietal pleura lining the left and right upper lobes.

Question 17:

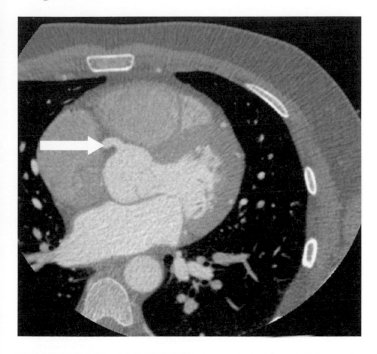

Name the arrowed structure	

■ Question 17: Axial CT of the heart

Answer: Right coronary artery

- The right coronary artery arises from the right coronary sinus (also known as the anterior sinus) and descends in the anterior atrioventricular groove.
- It has two major branches: the right marginal artery and, in about 60% of the population, the posterior descending artery (PDA).
- When the right coronary artery gives rise to the PDA, this is known as right dominance because the PDA supplies the posterior and lateral wall of the left ventricle.
- The right coronary artery supplies the right atrium, most of the right ventricle, and the inferior part of the left ventricle.
- It also supplies the sinoatrial node in approximately 60% of people and the atrioventricular node in approximately 80% of the population.

▪ Question 18:

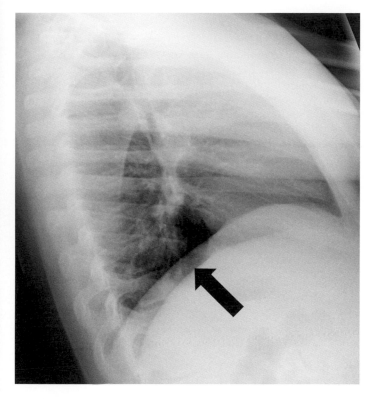

Name the arrowed structure	

▪ Question 18: Lateral chest radiograph

Answer: Left hemidiaphragm

- The diaphragm is a 2-3 mm thick highly convex muscle that forms the floor of the thoracic cage. It consists of a dome-shaped central tendon surrounded by sheets of striated muscle that attach to three groups of muscles or 'slips': the costal, sternal, and lumbar slips.
- It is easy to distinguish the left hemidiaphragm from the right on a lateral chest radiograph.
- The right hemidiaphragm can be seen in its entirety from the costophrenic recess posteriorly to the anterior aspect of the thorax. It is also usually higher than the left hemidiaphragm.
- Conversely, only part of the left hemidiaphragm is visible on a lateral radiograph. The outline of the left hemidiaphragm extends from the costophrenic recess to the back of the cardiac shadow.

Question 19:

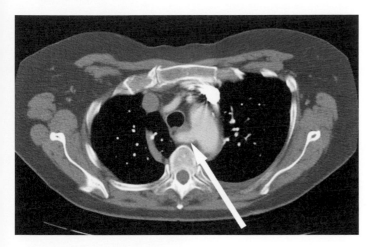

Name the arrowed structure	

Question 20:

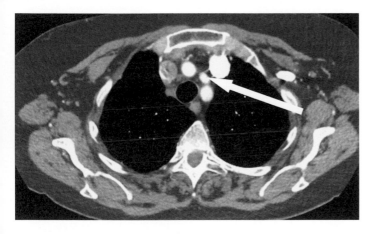

Name the arrowed structure	

▪ Question 19: Axial CT of the chest

Answer: Aberrant right subclavian artery

- The aberrant right subclavian artery is the most common of the arch vessel anomalies with an incidence of 0.5%.
- It usually arises distal to the left subclavian artery and passes posterior to the oesophagus before travelling to the right upper limb.
- Normally, no vessels pass posterior to the oesophagus.

▪ Question 20: Axial CT of the chest

Answer: Left common carotid artery

- The left common carotid artery is the second vessel to arise from the aortic arch.
- In the image, the left brachiocephalic vein is also filled with contrast medium because it has been injected via the left arm. It is important not to confuse it with one of the branches of the aorta. The brachiocephalic veins lie lateral to the three branches of the aortic arch.

Question 21:

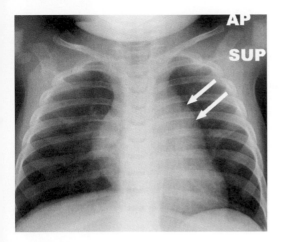

Name the arrowed structure	

■ Question 21: PA chest radiograph

Answer: Thymus

- The thymus is an anterior mediastinal structure situated anterior to the aorta and right ventricular outflow tract.
- It varies in size but, as a general rule, it is largest in children and adolescents where it is commonly bi-lobed or triangular in shape.
- This is one of the frequently occurring questions in the examination. Make sure to familiarise yourself with the variable appearances of the thymus in children.

Question 22:

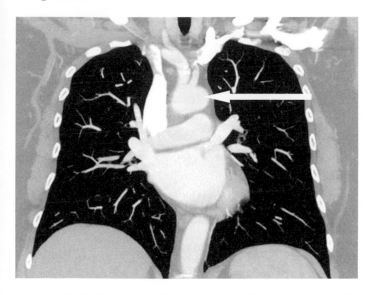

Name the arrowed structure	

Question 23:

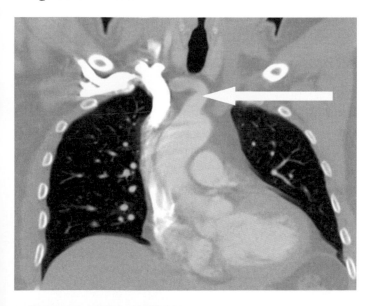

Name the arrowed structure	

▪ Question 22: Coronal CT of the chest (MIP image)

Answer: Arch of the aorta

- The arch of the aorta is the most superior aspect of the aorta.
- You can tell that this is the arch because within the thorax the only part of the aorta to have large vessels arising from it is the arch. These vessels supply the head, neck, and arms.

▪ Question 23: Coronal CT of the chest

Answer: The innominate artery (brachiocephalic artery)

- The innominate artery is the first branch of the aortic arch and shortly divides into the right common carotid and right subclavian arteries posterior to the right sternoclavicular joint.
- It is the largest and shortest of the arch vessels.

■ **Question 24:**

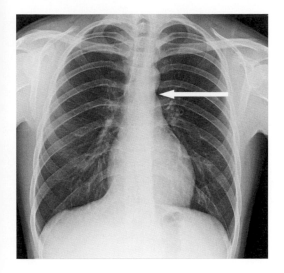

Name the arrowed structure	

■ Question 24: PA chest radiograph

Answer: Aortopulmonary window

- An aortopulmonary window is a radiological mediastinal space seen on frontal chest X-rays. It is a concave space that is bounded by the aortic arch superiorly and the left pulmonary artery inferiorly.
- It contains the ligamentum arteriosum, the left recurrent laryngeal nerve, lymph nodes, and fatty tissue.
- It is a common site for tumours and lymphadenopathy, in which case the concavity will be lost.

Question 25:

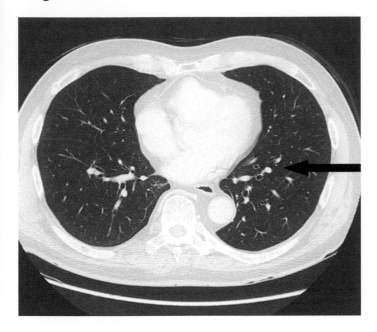

Name the arrowed structure	

▪ Question 25: Axial CT of the chest

Answer: Left lower lobe

- The left lower lobe has four segments: apical, anteromedial basal, lateral basal, and posterior basal segments.
- It is separated from the left upper lobe by the oblique fissure.

▪ Question 26:

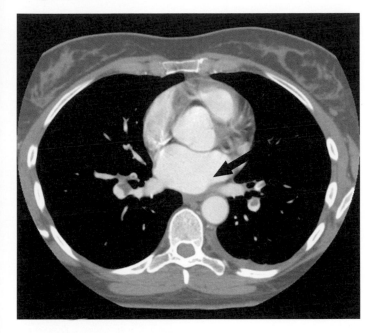

Name the arrowed structure	

▪ Question 27:

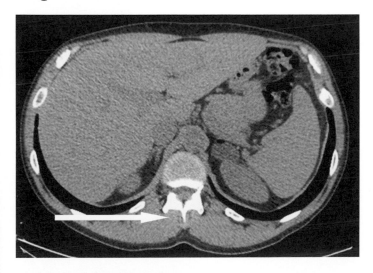

Name the arrowed structure	

■ Question 26: Axial CT of the chest

Answer: Left atrium

- The left atrium is the most posterior of the four cardiac chambers and lies close to the bodies of the thoracic vertebrae.
- The four pulmonary veins bring oxygenated blood to this chamber.
- The oesophagus is related to the posterior left atrial margin, which explains the incidence of dysphagia with left atrial enlargement.
- It may be of interest to note that there are bilateral pulmonary emboli in the image. However, you will not be shown any abnormalities in the examination.

■ Question 27: Axial CT of the abdomen

Answer: Right erector spinae muscle

- Erector spinae are a longitudinal set of three muscle fibres acting together as extensors of the spine.
- They arise from the crest of the sacrum and insert at various levels of the thoracic spine, cervical spine, and the base of the skull.
- On axial images, it is closely related to the vertebral column.

Question 28:

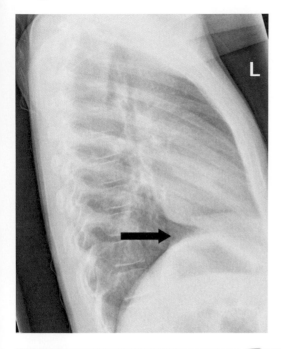

Name the arrowed structure	

■ Question 28: Lateral chest radiograph

Answer: Inferior vena cava

- The thoracic inferior vena cava (IVC) is an extremely short segment.
- On a lateral radiograph, the thoracic IVC occupies the posteroinferior corner of the posterior cardiac silhouette.
- The IVC can be difficult to delineate on a frontal chest radiograph. However, it forms part of the cardio-mediastinal silhouette where it occupies the right cardiophrenic angle.

Question 29:

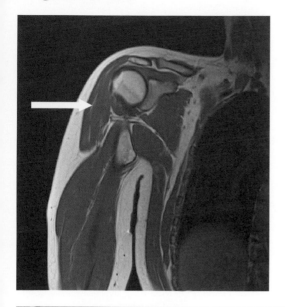

Name the arrowed structure	

Question 30:

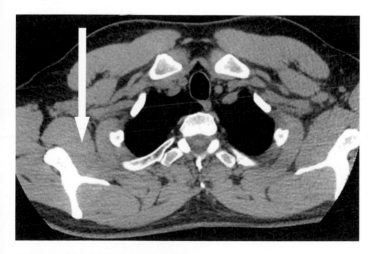

Name the arrowed structure	

▪ Question 29: Coronal MRI of the right arm

Answer: Right deltoid muscle

- The deltoid muscle is a strong abductor of the arm, consisting of three major groups of fibres: anterior, lateral, and posterior.
- The anterior fibres arise from the anterior border of the clavicle. The lateral fibres arise from the acromion process and the posterior fibres arise from the posterior aspect of the scapular spine.
- The deltoid fibres are distinctive in their strong but short, broad fibres, and the muscle is easily identifiable on CT reformats and MRI sequences. They insert at the deltoid tuberosity on the medial aspect of the humeral shaft.

▪ Question 30: Axial CT of the chest

Answer: Right subscapularis muscle

- The rotator cuff muscles are a favourite amongst examiners due to their clinical significance and their ability to discriminate candidates' anatomical knowledge.
- The subscapularis muscle—as the name implies—lines the subscapular fossa.
- On an axial reformat, it demonstrates an intimate anteromedial relation to the scapula.
- Unlike the other rotator cuff muscles, it inserts onto the lesser tubercle of the humerus anteriorly.

■ Question 31:

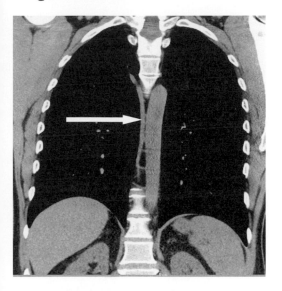

Name the arrowed structure	

■ Question 31: Coronal CT of the chest

Answer: The azygos vein

- The azygos vein is a small calibre vein that ascends from the level of T12 and arches over the right main bronchus to drain into the superior vena cava.
- It ascends just to the right of the vertebral column—as opposed to the hemiazygos and accessory hemi-azygos veins, which ascend to the left of the vertebral column.
- The azygos vein drains the posterior chest and abdominal walls.
- The azygos and hemiazygos veins may be very large if there is congenital atresia or obstruction of the inferior vena cava.

Question 32:

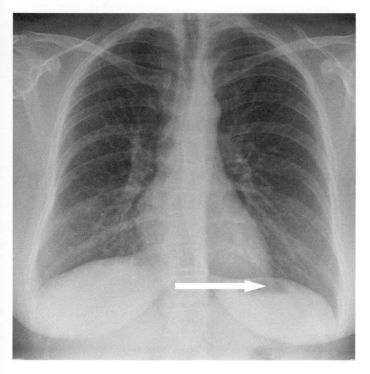

Name the arrowed structure	

■ Question 32: PA chest radiograph

Answer: Stomach bubble

- The stomach bubble is air in the fundus of the stomach.
- The bubble of air will be seen below the left hemidiaphragm if the patient is erect.
- It is useful to recognise this because, if the bubble is on the right, it provides a clue that the patient has situs inversus.

▪ Question 33:

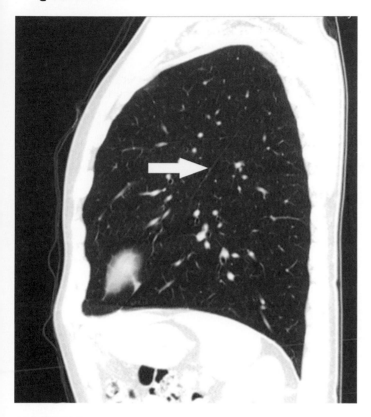

Name the arrowed structure	

▪ Question 33: Sagittal CT of the chest

Answer: Left oblique fissure

- The left oblique fissure separates the left upper lobe from the left lower lobe and extends from T4/T5 posteriorly in an anteroinferior direction to make contact with the diaphragm; as such, it is not seen on the frontal chest X-ray.
- The left oblique fissure is more vertically oriented than the right.
- If you are struggling to determine whether this is the left hemithorax or the right, count the number of lobes visible. On the right, there will be three lobes, and on the left, as in this case, there will be two.

▪ Question 34:

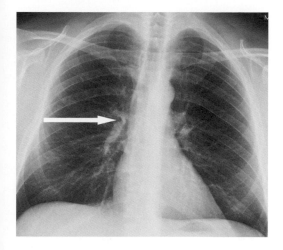

Name the arrowed structure	

■ Question 34: PA chest radiograph

Answer: Right hilar point

- The hilar point is the crossing point between the lower lobe pulmonary artery and the upper lobe pulmonary vein. The right hilar point lies at the level of the right 6th rib in the mid-axillary line.
- The left hilum is approximately 1 cm higher than the right. This is because the main pulmonary artery on the right passes anterior to the right main bronchus, whereas the left main pulmonary artery passes posteriorly and hooks over the left main bronchus.
- The hilar points are at the same level in approximately 5% of normal chest X-rays.
- The hilar angle is the angle between the two vessels and is normally 120°.

Question 35:

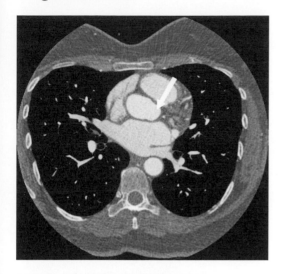

Name the arrowed structure	

■ Question 35: Axial contrast-enhanced CT of the chest

Answer: Left posterior sinus of Valsalva or left coronary sinus

- There are three sinuses of Valsalva:
  - Anterior or right coronary sinus
  - Left posterior or left coronary sinus
  - Right posterior or noncoronary sinus
- The sinuses are areas of focal dilation directly above the cusp of each valve.
- The right and left main coronary arteries arise from the right and left coronary sinuses, respectively. As the name suggests, no coronary artery arises from the noncoronary sinus.

Question 36:

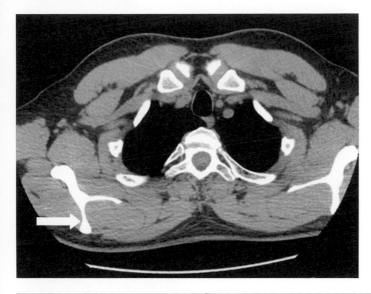

Name the arrowed structure	

■ Question 36: Axial CT of the chest

Answer: Right scapular spine

- The scapular spine is a bony plate arising obliquely from the posterior aspect of the scapula that separates the supraspinatus fossa from the infraspinatus fossa.
- The scapular spine extends superolaterally to end in a bony process, the acromion.

■ Question 37:

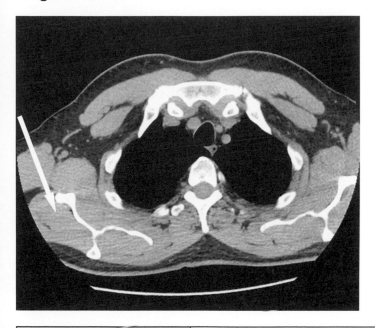

Name the arrowed structure	

■ Question 38:

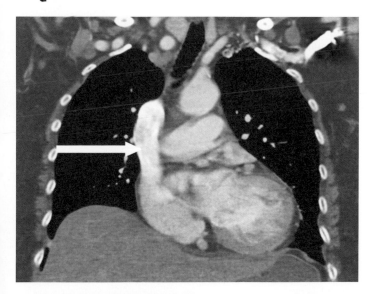

Name the arrowed structure	

■ Question 37: Axial CT of the chest

Answer: Right infraspinatus muscle

- The infraspinatus muscle is another member of the rotator cuff. As the name implies, the infraspinatus muscle occupies the infraspinatus fossa and inserts onto the greater tuberosity of the humerus.
- On axial CT, the infraspinatus muscle is separated from the supraspinatus by the spine of the scapula. The infraspinatus is lateral to the spine.
- The infraspinatus is also larger than the supraspinatus, which is another distinguishing feature.

■ Question 38: Coronal CT of the chest

Answer: Superior vena cava

- The superior vena cava (SVC) begins at the confluence of the right and left brachiocephalic veins. The latter usually runs obliquely from the left acromioclavicular joint to the right sternomanubrial junction.
- The SVC enters the right atrium at approximately the level of T3. Knowledge of this level is important to gauge whether central venous catheters are appropriately sited.

Question 39:

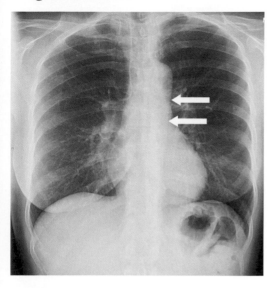

Name the arrowed structure	

■ Question 39: PA chest radiograph

Answer: Descending aorta

- The descending thoracic aorta is identifiable on the frontal and lateral projections of the chest radiograph.
- On the frontal projection, the lateral border of the descending aorta is seen behind the heart and lateral to the vertebral bodies.
- On the lateral projection, the descending aorta is seen less clearly overlying the thoracic spine.

▪ Question 40:

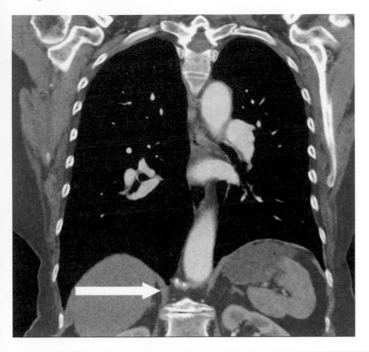

Name the arrowed structure	

■ Question 40: Coronal CT of the chest

Answer: Right diaphragmatic crus

- The diaphragmatic crura are strong tendinous structures that attach the diaphragm to the lumbar spine.
- They extend from the diaphragm in an inferomedial direction to attach to the vertebral column.
- The right crus is longer and extends to L3, whereas the left crus extends to L2.

▪ Question 41:

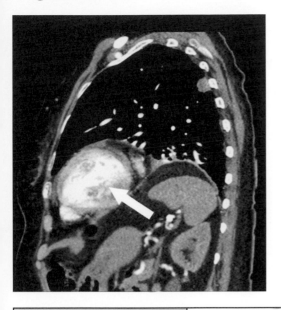

Name the arrowed structure	

▪ Question 41: Sagittal CT of the chest

Answer: Left ventricle

- You can tell that the image shows the left side of the chest because the spleen can be seen on the same slice.
- You can also tell that it is the ventricle rather than the atrium because of its anterior location within the thorax.
- Incidentally, there is a pulmonary nodule anterior to the 5th rib on this image that was found to be a metastasis.

Question 42:

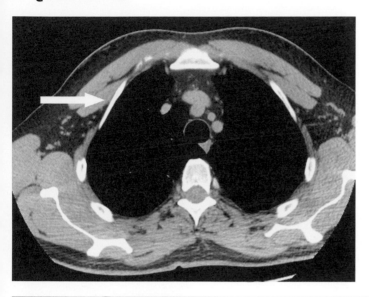

Name the arrowed structure	

▪ Question 42: Axial CT of the chest

Answer: Right pectoralis minor muscle

- The pectoralis minor muscle is a small, triangular anterior chest wall muscle that lies deep to the pectoralis major muscle.
- It has an insertion point (the apex of the triangle) at the coracoid process and attachments (the base) at 3rd, 4th, and 5th ribs with variation in the site of attachment.
- It acts as a scapular stabiliser and an accessory respiratory muscle by elevating the ribs during deep respiratory efforts.

Question 43:

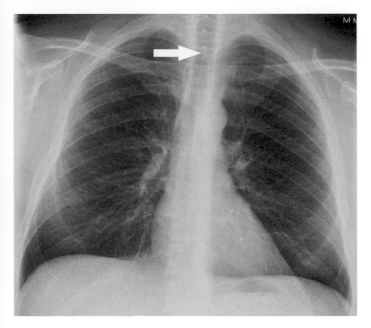

Name the arrowed structure	

■ Question 43: PA chest radiograph

Answer: T3 spinous process

- The spinous process is a bony prominence that is the midline coalescence of the two laminae.
- It is directed posteriorly and inferiorly at all levels and acts as an attachment for muscles and ligaments.
- The vertical distance between the spinous processes should be uniform. An abnormally increased or decreased distance is suspicious for a fracture or dislocation of the facet joints.

■ Question 44:

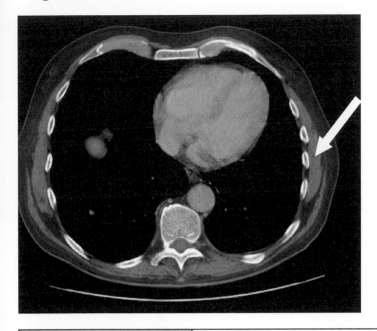

Name the arrowed structure	

▪ Question 44: Axial CT of the chest

Answer: Left serratus anterior muscle

- Serratus anterior forms the medial wall of the axilla and overlies the lateral thoracic wall.
- It inserts at the lateral wall of the scapula and is derived from broad muscular slips that arise from the first eight or nine ribs. This allows the muscle to act as a strong protractor of the scapula. It also assists in normal respiratory efforts (when the scapula is fixed).

▪ Question 45:

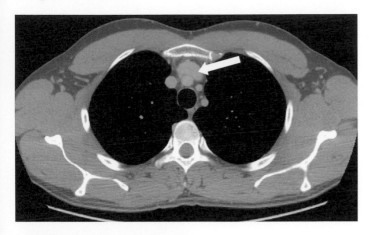

Name the arrowed structure	

▪ Question 46:

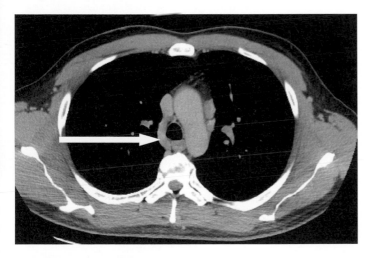

Name the arrowed structure	

▪ Question 45: Axial CT of the chest

Answer: Left brachiocephalic vein

- The left brachiocephalic vein has its origin from the union of the left internal jugular vein and the left subclavian vein.
- It is responsible for draining the head and neck and the left upper limb to the right atrium.
- It has a longer course than the right brachiocephalic vein and can be seen on axial CT slices coursing obliquely behind the sternum and anterior to the aortic arch branches to drain into the superior vena cava.

▪ Question 46: Axial CT of the chest

Answer: Azygos vein

- Following its vertical ascent lateral to the right side of the vertebral bodies, the azygos vein rises over the root of the right lung to join the superior vena cava as seen here.

Question 47:

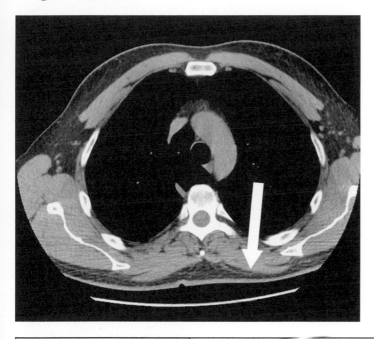

Name the arrowed structure	

▪ Question 47: Axial CT of the chest

Answer: Left trapezius muscle

- The trapezius muscle, so named for its trapezoidal shape, is a large superficial muscle of the back that has upper, middle, and lower fibres.
- The upper fibres attach to the vertebral column and the skull, whereas the middle and lower fibres attach to the spinous processes of C7 to T12.
- It inserts at the lateral aspects of the clavicle and scapula. It is the most superficial muscle of the back on axial slices.

Question 48:

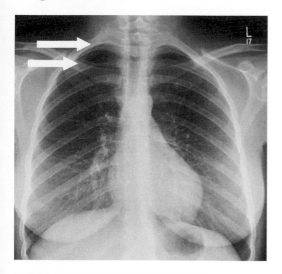

Name the arrowed structure	

■ Question 48: PA chest radiograph

Answer: Right cervical rib

- A cervical rib is an extra rib that arises from the transverse process of C7.
- It can be a bony or fibrous band.
- It occurs in 1 to 2% of the population. Cervical ribs are bilateral in 50% of cases.
- To distinguish this from a normal first rib, look at the transverse process from which it arises. A normal first thoracic rib will arise from an upward-sloping transverse process because the transverse processes of the thoracic vertebrae are always orientated in a superior direction. Conversely, the transverse processes of the cervical vertebrae are downward-sloping.

Question 49:

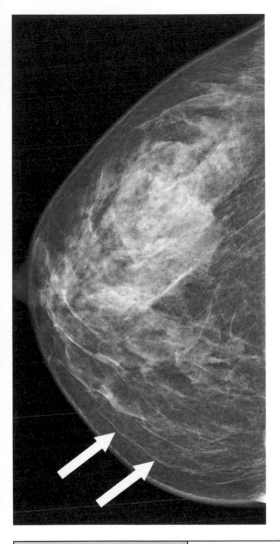

Name the arrowed structure	

■ Question 49: Mammogram

Answer: Cooper ligament or suspensory ligament

- The Cooper ligament is composed of fibrous bands of connective tissue that support the glandular part of the breast.
- Anteriorly, they attach to the skin and, posteriorly, to the fascia of the pectoralis major muscle.

▪ Question 50:

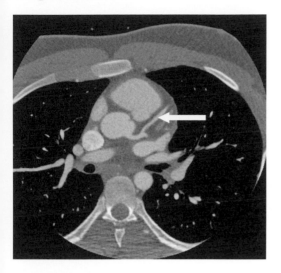

Name the arrowed structure	

■ Question 50: Axial contrast-enhanced CT of the chest

Answer: Left anterior descending artery

- Cardiac structures are much easier to identify and interpret on modern 64-slice CT scanners especially with the aid of electrocardiographic gating; therefore, it would be fair to ask a question about the coronary arteries.
- The left anterior descending artery (LAD) is one of two main branches of the left coronary artery, the other being the circumflex artery (the origin of which is visible on this image).
- The LAD descends in the anterior interventricular groove to the apex of the heart.
- It supplies blood to the left ventricle, interventricular groove, and occasionally to the right ventricle.

Chapter 3

Gastrointestinal, Gynaecological, and Urological Anatomy

Question 1:

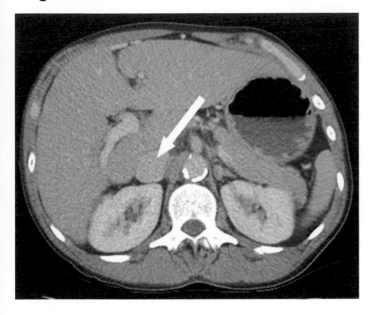

Name the arrowed structure	

Question 2:

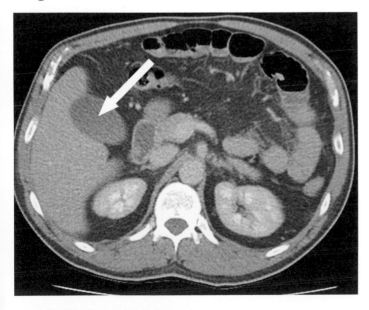

Name the arrowed structure	

▪ Question 1: Axial CT of the abdomen

Answer: Inferior vena cava

- The inferior vena cava (IVC) passes adjacent to to the posterior part of the liver.
- The IVC has a short intrathoracic course. This may be important when it comes to answering the question in the examination, 'intrathoracic inferior vena cava', if the marker points to the IVC above the diaphragm.
- In the image, the IVC is distended and appears larger than the aorta. Sometimes it can appear slitlike when it is collapsed; it varies with the phase of respiration and intravascular volume. Be sure to familiarise yourself with both appearances.
- A bilateral/double IVC is a well-described normal variant.

▪ Question 2: Axial CT of the abdomen

Answer: Gallbladder

- The gallbladder is a fluid-filled structure and therefore has a lower attenuation than the adjacent liver.
- Rarely, it may be intrahepatic, surrounded by liver parenchyma rather than on the undersurface of the liver.
- Its wall should be less than 3 mm in thickness.
- Gas within the gallbladder may be a normal finding shortly after sphincterotomy or biliary stent insertion.

■ Question 3:

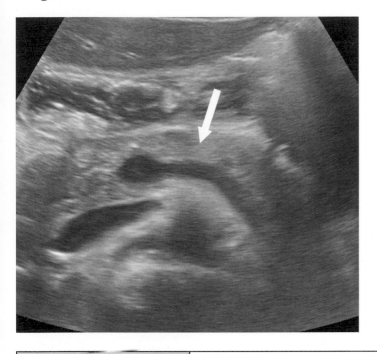

Name the arrowed structure	

■ Question 4:

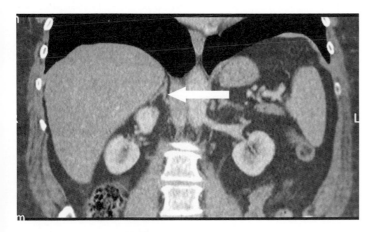

Name the arrowed structure	

▪ Question 3: US of the abdomen

Answer: Body of the pancreas

- The pancreas is divided into an uncinate process, head, neck, body, and tail.
- Only the neck has an anatomical definition; it is located anterior to the confluence of the superior mesenteric vein and splenic vein.

▪ Question 4: Coronal CT of the abdomen

Answer: Medial limb of the right adrenal gland

- The right adrenal gland is usually found cranial to the right kidney, whereas the left adrenal gland lies anteromedial to the upper pole of the left kidney.
- The normal thickness of a limb of the adrenal gland is approximately the same thickness as the adjacent diaphragm.
- The adrenal gland is composed of the body and the medial and lateral limbs. If in doubt as to how specific you should be in the examination, you should provide more information and specify the part of the adrenal gland that is labeled.

Question 5:

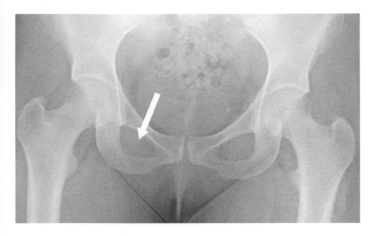

Name the arrowed structure	

Question 6:

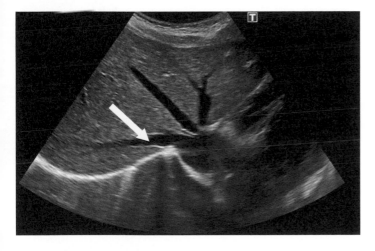

Name the arrowed structure	

■ Question 5: AP radiograph of the pelvis

Answer: Right obturator foramen

- The obturator foramen is bordered by the pubic rami and the ischial bone.
- The foramina are almost entirely covered by a ligamentous membrane.
- The obturator externus muscle originates from the external surface of the obturator membrane. The obturator internus muscle originates from the deep surface and hooks around the pelvic bones to insert onto the femur.

■ Question 6: Transverse US of the abdomen

Answer: Right hepatic vein

- The venous drainage of the liver is variable, but typically the majority of the liver is drained by three hepatic veins draining into the intrahepatic portion of the inferior vena cava (IVC).
- The caudate lobe drains directly into the IVC, which explains why this part of the liver is often not affected by disease processes in the same way as the remainder of the liver.
- The right hepatic vein is one of the landmarks used to separate segments V and VI as well as VII and VIII of the right lobe of the liver.

Question 7:

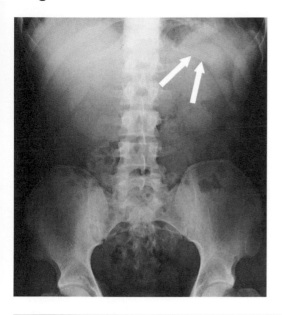

Name the arrowed structure	

■ Question 7: AP radiograph of the abdomen

Answer: Left 12th rib

- The 12th rib is one of the free floating ribs, which means that it is not attached anteriorly to the sternum.
- It can be seen on abdominal radiographs as the most inferior rib, tapering after a few centimetres.
- The 12th ribs can be helpful when counting the vertebral levels of the lumbar spine because their origin defines the T12 vertebral level.
- The 12th ribs can vary in length and may be absent.

Question 8:

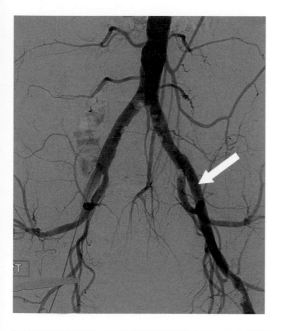

Name the arrowed structure	

■ Question 8: Angiogram of the iliac arteries

Answer: Left external iliac artery

- The common iliac arteries divide into the internal and external iliac arteries.
- The external iliac arteries run parallel and usually lateral to the external iliac veins.
- The external iliac artery becomes the femoral artery as it passes the inguinal ligament. This is a common pitfall in the examination.

Question 9:

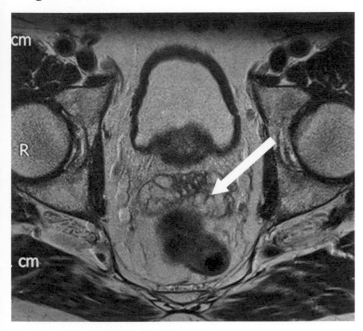

Name the arrowed structure	

Question 10:

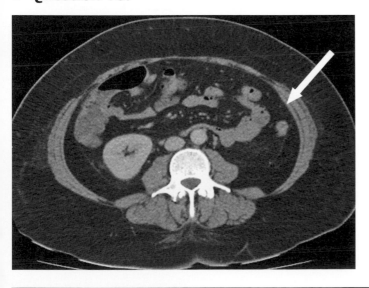

Name the arrowed structure	

▪ Question 9: Axial T2-weighted MRI of the male pelvis

Answer: Left seminal vesicle

- The seminal vesicles are paired structures posterior to the male bladder.
- Due to the high water content of the vesicles, they are of high signal intensity on T2-weighted MRIs.
- It is possible to confuse the seminal vesicles with ovaries when looking at just one slice. The way to determine whether this is a male or female pelvis is to look for the presence of the uterus—not here in this example—and to look for the presence of the prostate gland, situated behind the bladder as in this image.

▪ Question 10: Axial CT of the abdomen

Answer: Left transversus abdominis muscle

- The left transversus abdominis muscle is the innermost of the lateral abdominal muscles. Its fibres run transversely from lateral to medial.
- On its inferior border, it forms a tendinous fold, part of which is the roof of the inguinal canal.

Question 11:

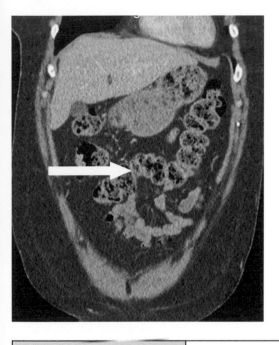

Name the arrowed structure	

■ Question 11: Coronal CT of the abdomen

Answer: Transverse colon

- The transverse colon is the most distal part of the colon to be supplied by branches from the superior mesenteric artery.
- It is suspended from the transverse mesocolon and lies within the peritoneal cavity.
- It is of variable length and may be seen drooping as far down as the pelvis.

Question 12:

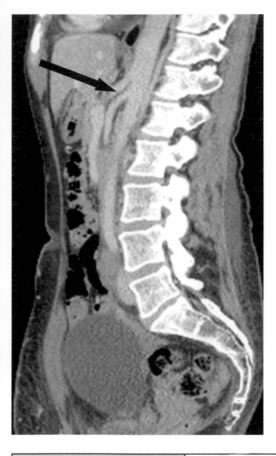

Name the arrowed structure	

■ Question 12: Sagittal CT of the abdomen and pelvis

Answer: Coeliac trunk

- The coeliac trunk is the first anterior branch of the abdominal aorta and supplies the foregut.
- It gives rise to the common hepatic, splenic, and left gastric arteries.

Question 13:

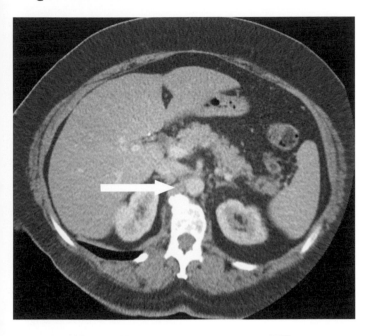

Name the arrowed structure	

■ Question 13: Axial CT of the abdomen

Answer: Right crus of the diaphragm

- The diaphragmatic crura are a paired structure; however, the right crus extends more inferiorly to L3 and may be confused with other structures.
- The left crus inserts onto L2.

Question 14:

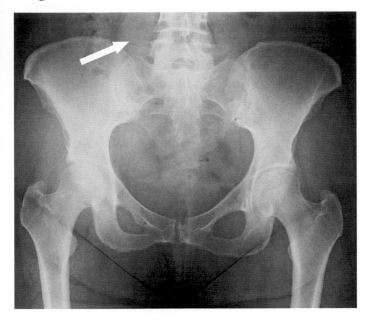

Name the arrowed structure	

Question 15:

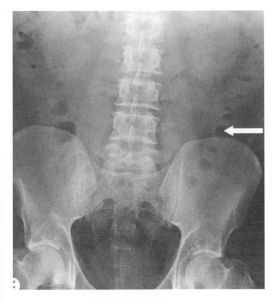

Name the arrowed structure	

▪ Question 14: AP radiograph of the pelvis

Answer: Right psoas major muscle

- The psoas major muscle may be seen on plain radiographs as an elongated, wedge-shaped density running obliquely next to the lumbar spine.
- It is one of the flexors of the hip, originating from the lateral border of the spine (T12 to L5) and inserting into the lesser trochanter of the femur.

▪ Question 15: AP radiograph of the abdomen

Answer: Descending colon

- The descending colon is often seen as a gas-filled structure on plain radiography, running in the superoinferior direction in the left flank.
- It can be identified as large bowel by its haustral pattern and faeces may be seen within.
- The upper limit of normal for the descending colon is 6 cm in diameter. The caecum may measure up to 9 cm and small bowel up to 3 cm.

Question 16:

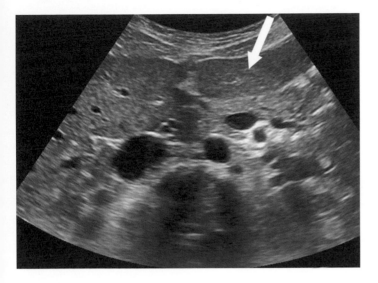

Name the arrowed structure	

▪ Question 16: Transverse US of the upper abdomen

Answer: Lateral segment of the left lobe of liver

- The functional left lobe of the liver lies to the left of the Cantlie line. This is the plane between th inferior vena cava (IVC) and the gallbladder fossa. The left lobe consists of segments I to IV—named b Couinaud.
- It crosses the midline and lies under the diaphragm with the heart superiorly, the stomach and duode num inferiorly, and aorta and IVC posteriorly.
- The left lobe is supplied by the left portal vein and left hepatic artery. Venous drainage is by the le hepatic vein, and biliary drainage is via the left hepatic duct.
- At first glance, the image is disorientating because only a part of the left and right lobes of the live can be seen. However, if you look at the rest of the image, you will notice the IVC and aorta are sittin anterior to the vertebral body in the bottom central part of the image. You will also notice the fissure fo the falciform ligament, which divides the left lobe into medial and lateral segments. More deeply is th pancreas, which is more reflective than the liver, and the splenic vein posteriorly.
- The figure below shows the segments of the liver as described by Couinaud.

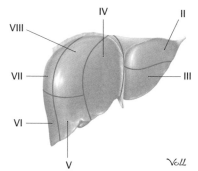

From Atlas of Anatomy, © Thieme 2008,
illustration by Markus Voll.

Question 17:

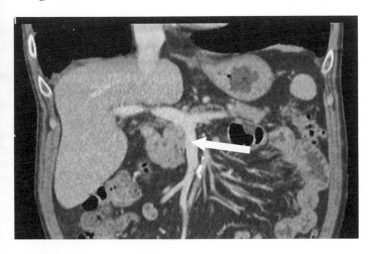

Name the arrowed structure	

Question 18:

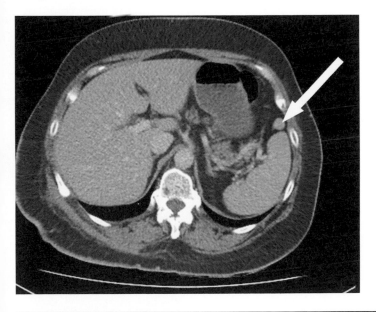

Name the arrowed structure	

■ Question 17: Coronal CT of the abdomen

Answer: Superior mesenteric vein

- The superior mesenteric vein (SMV) is the principal venous drainage of the bowel. It joins the splenic vein to form the portal vein.
- The SMV runs to the right of the superior mesenteric artery (SMA). Reversal of the SMA/SMV relationship is a feature of intestinal malrotation.
- The confluence of the SMV and splenic vein defines the neck of the pancreas.

■ Question 18: Axial CT of the abdomen

Answer: Splenunculus

- Splenunculus is a very common normal variant that can be confused with disease such as lymphadenopathy.
- It is often seen as a small, rounded structure near the hilum of the spleen of isointensity/equal reflectivity/isodensity to the spleen on MRI/US/CT, respectively.
- A splenunculus should follow the enhancement characteristics of the spleen in all phases of enhancement.

▪ Question 19:

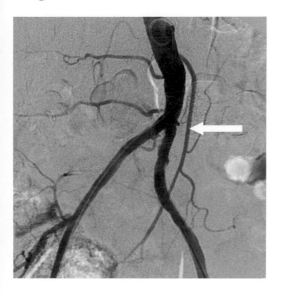

Name the arrowed structure	

▪ Question 19: Aortic angiogram

Answer: Inferior mesenteric artery

- The inferior mesenteric artery is the third unpaired branch of the aorta.
- It is a much smaller calibre vessel compared with the coeliac trunk or superior mesenteric artery.
- It supplies blood to the mid transverse colon through to the proximal rectum.
- Branches of the internal iliac artery supply the middle and distal rectum and anal canal.
- The watershed area is the region of colon between the supply of the superior mesenteric artery and inferior mesenteric artery, and is more vulnerable to ischaemia.

Question 20:

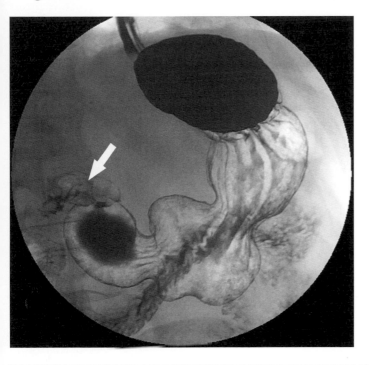

Name the arrowed structure	

▪ Question 20: Barium meal

Answer: Duodenal cap

- The duodenal cap is the first part of the duodenum and the only intraperitoneal section of the duodenum.
- It is approximately 2.5 cm in length.
- The duodenum extends from the pylorus to the jejunum. Four segments make up its length (D1, 2, 3, and 4).

Question 21:

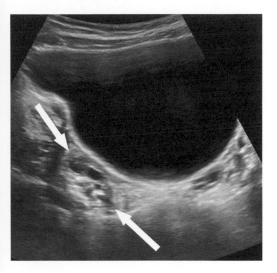

Name the arrowed structure	

■ Question 21: Transabdominal US of the pelvis

Answer: Right ovary

- The ovaries are usually found lateral to the uterus and measure approximately 2 × 2 × 3 cm.
- The bladder acts as an acoustic window to allow better visualisation of the pelvic structures, as well as pushing gas-filled bowel out of the way.
- The ovaries are better visualised with a transvaginal US.

▪ Question 22:

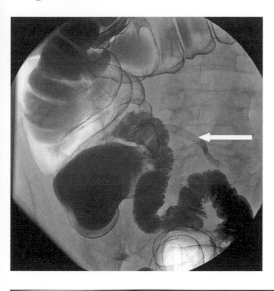

Name the arrowed structure	

▪ Question 23:

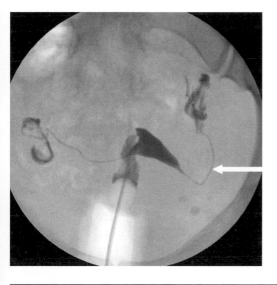

Name the arrowed structure	

■ Question 22: Barium enema

Answer: Appendix

- The appendix is a blind ending loop of bowel that arises from the caecum. It is usually seen in the right lower quadrant.
- On a fluoroscopic study such as this barium enema, the appendix may appear as a contrast medium–filled structure or, as in this case, there is double contrast, with gas in the lumen and contrast medium lining the appendix wall.
- The appendix and a Meckel diverticulum are the only blind ending structures that can be seen on a normal barium examination.

■ Question 23: Hysterosalpingogram

Answer: Left fallopian tube

- If you have not seen a hysterosalpingogram before, you may have difficulty identifying the fallopian tubes. On the left of the image, you can see the inferior sacroiliac joint and the pelvic brim; therefore, you know it is a pelvic structure.
- On this AP view, the uterus is seen as a triangular, contrast-filled structure with the fallopian tubes arising from each cornua.
- Contrast medium is seen through the length of the fallopian tubes and within the peritoneum where it flows out through the ampulla (the widened structures at the end of the fallopian tubes).

Question 24:

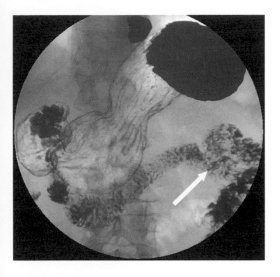

Name the arrowed structure	

Question 25:

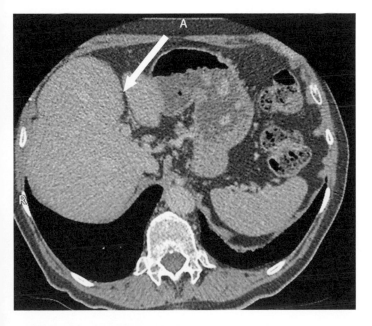

Name the arrowed structure	

▪ Question 24: Barium meal

Answer: Jejunum

- The jejunum makes up the proximal two fifths of the small bowel. It has a characteristic feathery appearance in contrast to the relatively featureless ileum.
- It begins at the duodenojejunal flexure at the level of L2 and extends to the ileum.
- It has a wider lumen, thicker wall, and more prominent valvulae conniventes than the ileum.

▪ Question 25: Axial CT of the abdomen

Answer: Fissure of falciform ligament

- The falciform ligament is attached to the diaphragm and separates the medial and lateral segments of the left lobe of the liver.
- The falciform ligament is composed of two layers of peritoneum closely united together.
- Inferiorly, the falciform ligament contains the round ligament (the obliterated umbilical vein) between its layers.
- The round ligament (also known as the ligamentum teres) is found on the inferior aspect of the liver anterior to the caudate lobe.
- It merges with the fissure of the ligamentum venosum, which contains the obliterated ductus venosus that connects the left portal vein to the left hepatic vein.

▪ Question 26:

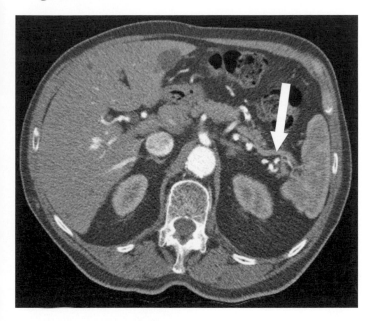

Name the arrowed structure	

▪ Question 27:

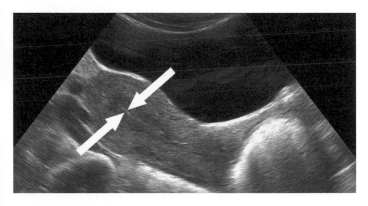

Name the arrowed structure	

▪ Question 26: Axial CT of the abdomen

Answer: Splenic vein

- The splenic vein runs alongside the splenic artery and the pancreas to form the portal vein at its confluence with the superior mesenteric vein.
- Differentiation from the splenic artery can be difficult. It is useful to consider the intravenous contrast phase of the scan. In this study, the contrast is in the arterial phase (because the aorta is enhanced). Therefore, the splenic artery will be bright, whereas the vein will be of lower attenuation.
- As the splenic artery is tortuous, it is rarely imaged whole in one axial slice.

▪ Question 27: Longitudinal US of the pelvis

Answer: Endometrium

- The endometrium is the inner lining of the uterus.
- On ultrasound, it can be recognised as a thin, hyperreflective layer.
- In a premenopausal woman, the thickness of the endometrium is dependent on the menstrual cycle but should be < 15 mm.
- The upper limit of normal is 10 mm in an asymptomatic postmenopausal woman. In a postmenopausal woman with bleeding, an endometrial thickness of greater than 4 mm will warrant further investigation.
- The uterus has a thicker outer muscular layer called the myometrium.

Question 28:

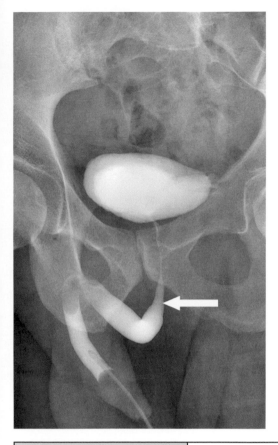

Name the arrowed structure	

▪ Question 28: Male urethrogram

Answer: Bulbar urethra

- There are not many structures that could have this appearance, so even if you have never seen a urethrogram before, you should be able to guess.
- There are four parts to the male urethra: penile, bulbar, membranous, and prostatic. The membranous urethra is the narrowest.

Question 29:

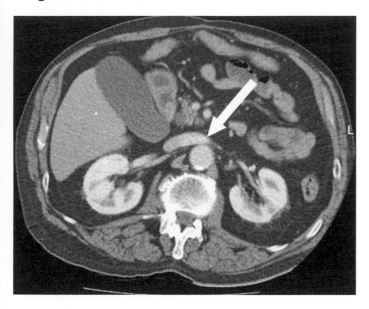

Name the arrowed structure	

Question 30:

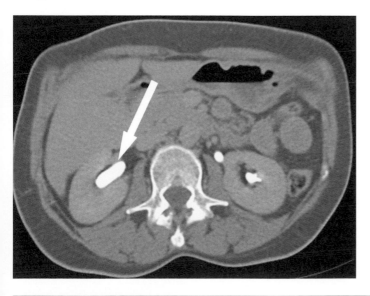

Name the arrowed structure	

■ Question 29: Axial CT of the abdomen

Answer: Left renal vein

- The left renal vein is longer than the right renal vein and crosses under the origin of the superior mesenteric artery.
- The left renal vein usually crosses anterior to the aorta.
- It may, however, pass behind the aorta (a retroaortic left renal vein) or have elements anterior and posterior to the aorta (a circumaortic left renal vein). When present, the retroaortic component is always caudal to the preaortic component.

■ Question 30: Axial CT urogram

Answer: Right ureter

- There is usually one ureter on either side, but they can be double in duplex kidneys.
- Ureters are easy to see on delayed phase renal scans (usually acquired more than 10 minutes after intravenous contrast medium injection).
- As the kidneys do not lie at the same level, one ureter may be seen in cross section while the other ureter is imaged at the level of the renal pelvis. Excreted intravenous contrast within the ureter may help to identify it.

▪ Question 31:

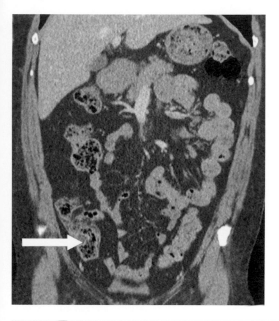

Name the arrowed structure	

■ Question 31: Coronal CT of the abdomen and pelvis

Answer: Caecum

- The caecum is the first part of the colon.
- It becomes the ascending colon just superior to the ileocaecal junction.
- The appendix can often be seen arising from the caecum proximal to the ileocaecal junction.
- The caecum is a common site of disease and should always be reviewed. The maximum diameter on an abdominal radiograph is 9 cm.

Question 32:

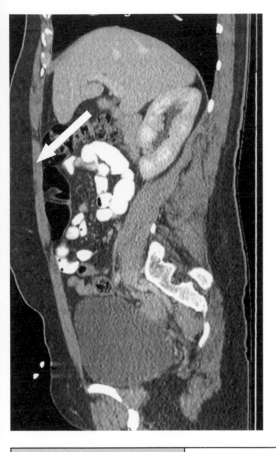

Name the arrowed structure	

▪ Question 32: Sagittal CT of the abdomen and pelvis

Answer: Rectus abdominis muscle

- The rectus abdominis are paired anterior abdominal wall muscles. They consist of multiple muscle bellies with intervening tendinous intersections.
- In the midline, the two muscles are separated by a tendinous structure called the linea alba. This is where the aponeuroses of the lateral abdominal muscles insert.

Question 33:

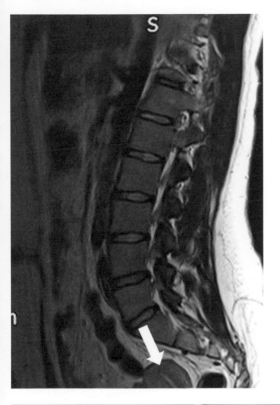

Name the arrowed structure	

▪ Question 33: Sagittal T2-weighted MRI of the lumbar spine and sacrum

Answer: Fundus of uterus

- The uterus lies between the bladder and rectum. It consists of the fundus, body, and cervix.
- The uterus has a characteristic layered appearance, especially on MRI and ultrasound.
- Endometrial thickness varies with age and stage of menstrual cycle. The upper limit of normal in an asymptomatic postmenopausal women is 10 mm.
- In the examination, it is quite common to be asked to name a structure that is not part of the main structures being imaged, so-called 'edge of film' structures.

Question 34:

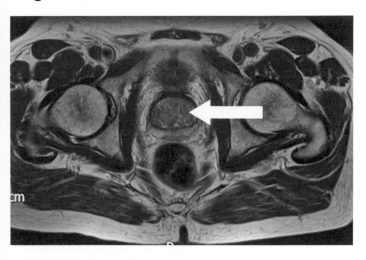

Name the arrowed structure	

Question 35:

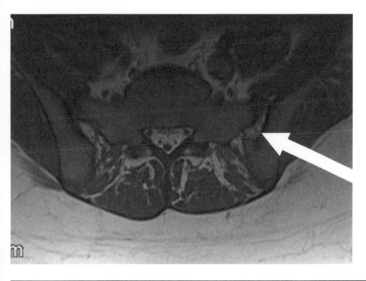

Name the arrowed structure	

■ Question 34: Axial T2-weighted MRI of the male pelvis

Answer: Prostate gland

- The prostate gland is a walnut-sized gland in the male pelvis, lying at the apex of the urinary bladder.
- The urethra passes in the superoinferior direction.
- The normal prostate gland has a characteristic zonal anatomy on T2-weighted MR imaging, consisting of a transitional, central, and peripheral zone as well as the anterior fibromuscular stroma.

■ Question 35: Axial T1-weighted MRI of the sacrum

Answer: Left sacroiliac joint

- The sacroiliac joint is a large, partly fibrous, partly synovial joint between the sacral ala and the iliac bone.
- It is stabilised by very strong ligaments.

■ Question 36:

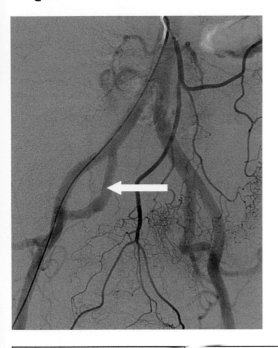

Name the arrowed structure	

■ Question 36: Iliac angiogram

Answer: Right internal iliac artery

- The common iliac artery bifurcates into the internal and external iliac arteries.
- The internal iliac artery has a posterior course compared to the anterior course of the external iliac artery.
- The internal iliac artery supplies blood to the pelvic viscera and muscles.
- There are two divisions of the internal iliac artery: anterior and posterior.
- Branches of the anterior division are the umbilical artery, obturator artery, inferior vesical artery, middle rectal artery, vaginal artery, uterine artery, internal pudendal artery, and the inferior gluteal artery.
- Branches of the posterior division are the superior gluteal artery, iliolumbar artery, and the lateral sacral artery.

▪ Question 37:

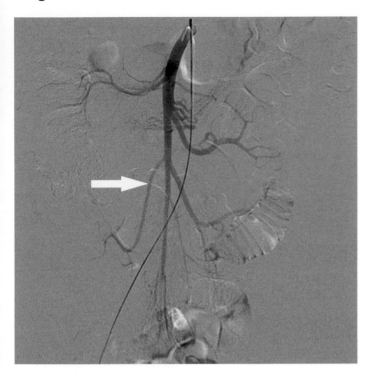

Name the arrowed structure	

■ Question 37: Superior mesenteric angiogram

Answer: Ileocolic artery

- The superior mesenteric artery supplies blood to the entire small intestines (foregut) and colon from the caecum through to the mid-transverse colon (midgut).
- The ileocolic artery supplies the caecum, appendix, and proximal ascending colon.
- The branches of the superior mesenteric artery, in a clockwise manner, are as follows:

Artery	Distribution
Inferior pancreatico-duodenal artery	Head of pancreas and distal duodenum
Jejunal branches	Jejunum
Ileal branches	Ileum
Ileocolic	Caecum, appendix, and proximal ascending colon
Right colic	Ascending colon (except proximal section)
Middle colic	Transverse colon (up to midpoint)

- The terminal superior mesenteric artery is seen in the midline of this angiogram and anastomoses with the ileal branches.

■ **Question 38:**

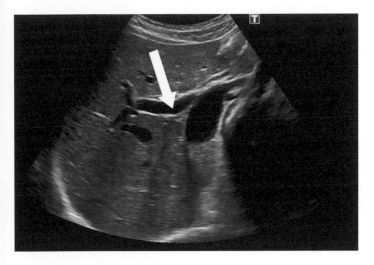

Name the arrowed structure	

▪ Question 38: Longitudinal US of the liver

Answer: Portal vein

- The portal vein originates at the confluence of the splenic vein and the superior mesenteric vein.
- It provides the liver with the majority of its blood supply, entering the liver at the porta hepatis together with the hepatic artery and the common bile duct. The portal vein bifurcates and supplies the left and right lobes of the liver.
- The flow in the splenic vein is hepatopetal—toward the liver.
- The portal vein and its branches typically have 'bright' (reflective) walls, which distinguishes them from the hepatic veins, which do not have reflective walls.

Question 39:

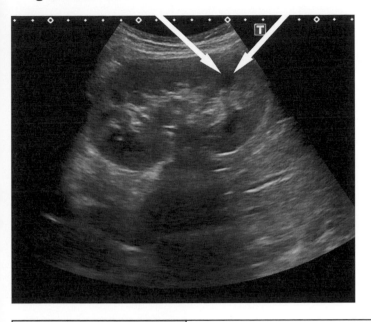

Name the arrowed structure	

▪ Question 39: Longitudinal US of the kidney

Answer: Renal pyramid

- The kidneys have renal pyramids that are conical structures with renal cortex externally and renal medulla internally.
- The renal papilla is at the apex of the pyramid and is part of the collecting system of the kidney.
- Fetal lobulation may persist in the adult, which makes the pyramidal structure of the kidneys more obvious.

Question 40:

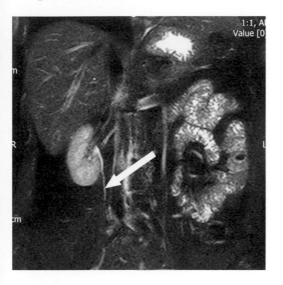

Name the arrowed structure	

▪ Question 40: Coronal T2-weighted MRI of the abdomen

Answer: Right ureter

- The ureter drains the renal collecting system and connects the kidney to the bladder.
- The ureter starts at the pelviureteric junction and ends at the vesicoureteric junction distally. These two points are common areas of obstruction.
- The ureters are lined by urothelium, which is prone to field change—the concept of multicentric cancer producing multiple transitional (urothelial) cell cancers.

Question 41:

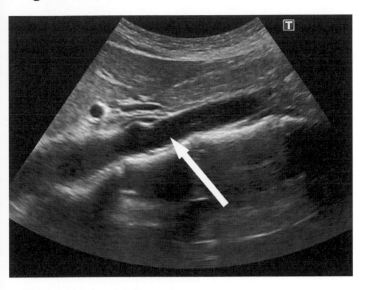

Name the arrowed structure	

Question 42:

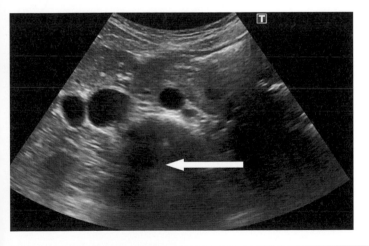

Name the arrowed structure	

▪ Question 41: US of the abdomen

Answer: Abdominal aorta

- The abdominal aorta can easily be assessed with ultrasound. It may be confused with the inferior vena cava, but only the aorta has anterior branches and lies to the left of the midline.
- The anteroposterior diameter of the normal aorta is < 3 cm.
- Colour Doppler can be used to assess the pulsatile arterial blood flow.

▪ Question 42: Transverse US of the abdomen

Answer: Vertebral body

- The vertebral body may be seen on US as a low reflectivity shadow.
- It lies posterior to the aorta and inferior vena cava.
- The spinal cord and theca can be seen as poorly reflective internal structures.
- Although not usually examined with US, the vertebral body is a common examination question because it is readily visible with US.

Question 43:

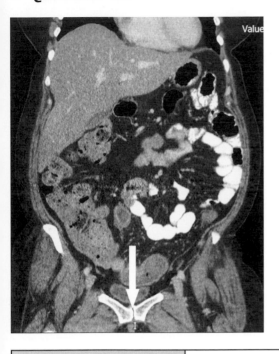

Name the arrowed structure	

■ Question 43: Coronal CT of the abdomen and pelvis

Answer: Symphysis pubis

- The symphysis pubis is a non-synovial cartilaginous joint in the midline between the paired pubic bones.
- The bladder lies immediately deep to the pubic symphysis.

Question 44:

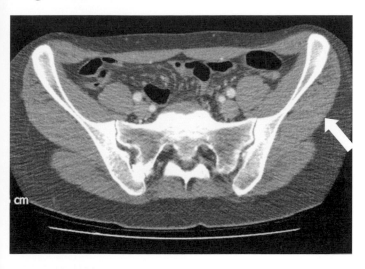

Name the arrowed structure	

Question 45:

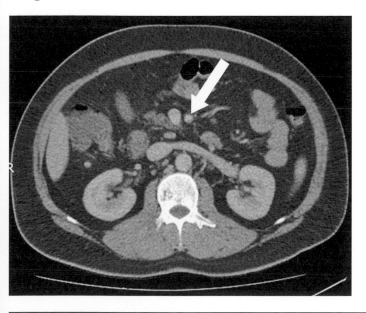

Name the arrowed structure	

▪ Question 44: Axial CT of the pelvis

Answer: Left gluteus medius muscle

• The gluteus medius muscle is the middle of the three gluteal muscles.
• Because gluteus maximus, the most superficial of the three muscles, originates more inferiorly, gluteus medius appears to be the most superficial in the superior sections of the pelvis, as on the image.
• It inserts distally on the anterolateral aspect of the greater trochanter of the femur.

▪ Question 45: Axial CT of the abdomen

Answer: Superior mesenteric artery

• The superior mesenteric artery is the second anterior branch of the abdominal aorta and supplies the midgut.
• It runs parallel to, and to the left of, the superior mesenteric vein (SMV). It enhances synchronously with the aorta in the arterial phase and may show calcification, which helps to distinguish it from the SMV in axial images.
• It passes anterior to the left renal vein, the third part of the duodenum, and the uncinate process of the pancreas.

■ Question 46:

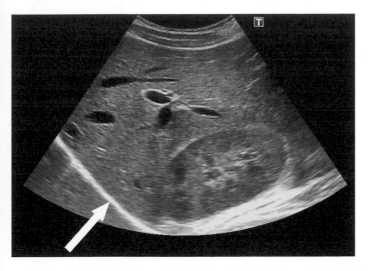

Name the arrowed structure	

■ Question 47:

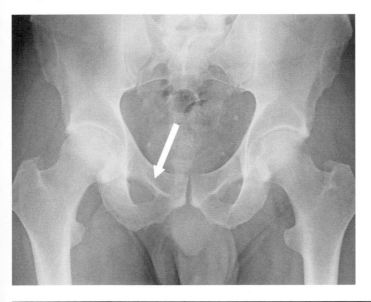

Name the arrowed structure	

■ Question 46: US of the liver

Answer: Right hemidiaphragm

- The diaphragm is a reflective, linear structure on US. It may be the source of reverberation artefacts on US.
- It is a dome-shaped sheet of muscle with a central membranous part.
- It is innervated by the C3-5 nerves. It separates the thorax from the abdomen and is pierced by the inferior vena cava (level T8), oesophagus (T10), and aorta (T12).
- Centrally, the crura of the diaphragm extend inferiorly along the lumbar spine.

■ Question 47: AP radiograph of the pelvis

Answer: Right superior pubic ramus

- The superior pubic ramus is one third of the pubic bone.
- It forms the superior border of the obturator foramen and the anterior aspect of the pelvic brim.
- Its superior surface is the continuation of the iliopectineal line and forms the insertion point for the pectineus muscle.

Question 48:

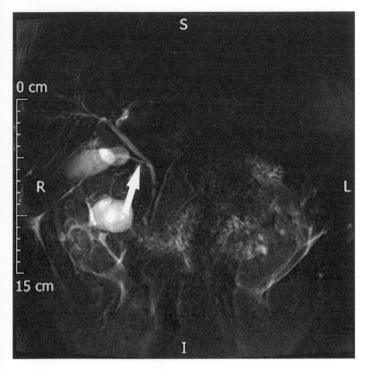

Name the arrowed structure	

▪ Question 48: MR cholangiopancreatogram

Answer: Cystic duct

- The cystic duct connects the gallbladder with the rest of the biliary tree.
- It is of variable length and joins the common hepatic duct to form the common bile duct at a variable point either proximally (close to the liver) or distally (near the pancreas). A low insertion is important to mention in reports because this has consequences for surgeons if they perform a cholecystectomy.

Question 49:

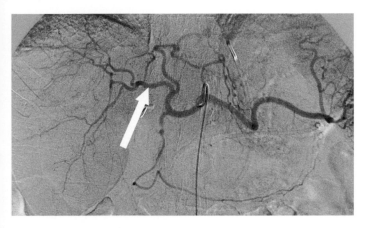

Name the arrowed structure	

■ Question 49: Coeliac angiogram

Answer: Right hepatic artery

- You can identify this as an angiogram of the coeliac axis by the long and tortuous splenic artery going to the spleen. The ribs in the left upper corner of the image tell you that it is the upper abdomen.
- The common hepatic artery divides into the right and left hepatic arteries, which supply the right and left lobes of the liver.
- Thirty percent of the blood supply to the liver is from the hepatic arteries. The other 70% is from the portal vein.
- There are a number of normal variants of the hepatic arteries of which to be aware. The common hepatic artery or the right hepatic artery can arise from the superior mesenteric artery instead of the coeliac trunk. The left hepatic artery can arise from the left gastric artery. It is also possible to have accessory hepatic arteries.

Question 50:

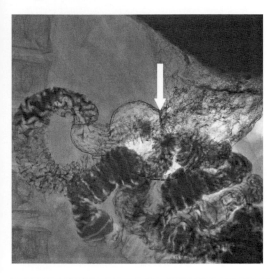

Name the arrowed structure	

■ Question 50: Barium meal

Answer: Incisura of lesser curvature

- The incisura is an angulation of the lesser curve of the stomach.
- It indicates the junction of the body and the antrum.

Chapter 4

Musculoskeletal Anatomy

■ Question 1:

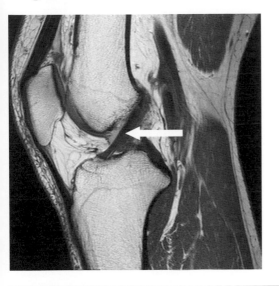

Name the arrowed structure	

■ Question 2:

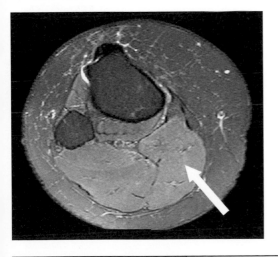

Name the arrowed structure	

▪ Question 1: Sagittal MRI of the knee

Answer: Anterior cruciate ligament

- The anterior cruciate ligament extends from the anterior intercondylar notch to the posteromedial aspect of the lateral femoral condyle.
- There are two bands: anteromedial and posterolateral.
- Their main function is to prevent posterior displacement of the tibia on flexion/extension.
- It is seen as a low intensity black band on T1-weighted/proton density MRI.
- However, it may just be the anteromedial band that appears black.

▪ Question 2: Axial MRI of the right lower leg

Answer: Medial head of the right gastrocnemius muscle

- The gastrocnemius muscle has two heads: the medial head arises from the medial condyle of the femur and the lateral head originates from the lateral condyle of the femur.
- The soleus and gastrocnemius muscle tendons join together to form the Achilles tendon, which inserts onto the calcaneus. The soleus and gastrocnemius muscles are known as the triceps surae.
- A sesamoid bone known as the fabella is commonly found in the lateral head of the gastrocnemius muscle.

▪ Question 3:

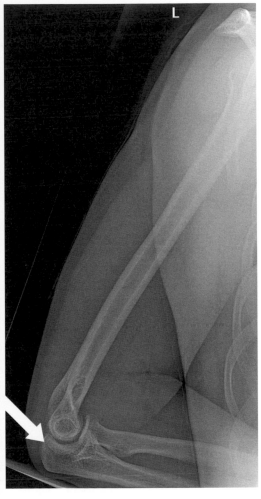

Name the arrowed structure	

▪ Question 3: Lateral radiograph of the left elbow

Answer: Olecranon process of ulna

- The proximal ulna articulates with the humerus via a hooklike projection with two curved eminences.
- The curved posterior eminence is the olecranon, which fits into the olecranon fossa of the humerus and articulates with the trochlea of the humerus.
- Make sure that you are able to distinguish between the olecranon and the coronoid process, which is the volar eminence of the proximal ulna.
- The triceps brachii muscle inserts onto the olecranon process.

Question 4:

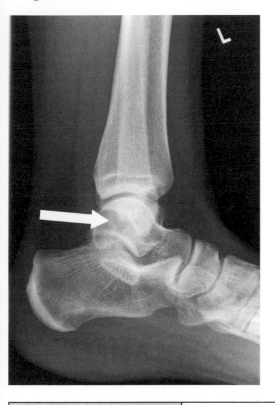

Name the arrowed structure	

▪ Question 4: Lateral radiograph of the left ankle

Answer: Left talus

- The talus can be divided into three parts: head, neck, and body.
- It articulates with the calcaneus caudally and navicular bone anteriorly.
- The tarsal sinus is a cylindrical cavity between the talus and calcaneus on the lateral aspect of the foot. It runs medially and opens posterior to the sustentaculum tali of the calcaneus.

Question 5:

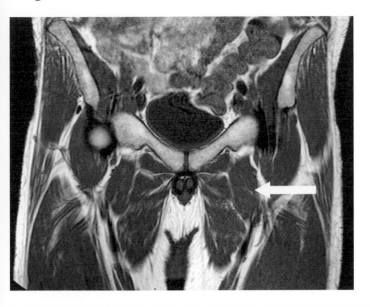

Name the arrowed structure	

Question 5: Coronal T1-weighted MRI of the pelvis

Answer: Left pectineus muscle

- The pectineus muscle adducts, flexes, and assists medial rotation of the thigh.
- It is an anterior muscle that attaches to the superior pubic ramus superiorly and the pectineal line of the femur (beneath the lesser trochanter) inferiorly.

Question 6:

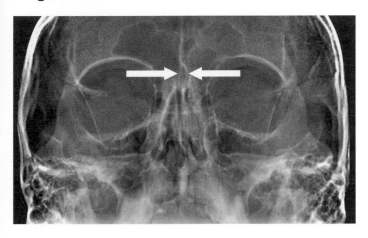

Name the arrowed structure	

Question 7:

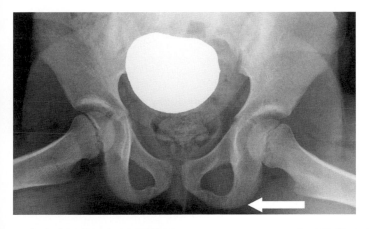

Name the arrowed structure	

▪ Question 6: Orbital radiograph

Answer: Crista galli

- *Crista galli* is Latin for 'crest of the cock'.
- On a frontal radiograph, the crista galli appears as a diamond-shaped bone in the midline at the level of the superior orbits.
- It arises from the cribriform plate of the ethmoid bone.
- It is the anterior attachment for the falx cerebri.

▪ Question 7: Frogleg lateral hip radiograph

Answer: Left ischial tuberosity

- On this radiograph, the ischial tuberosity is seen lateral to the inferior pubic ramus; however, in reality, it is much more posterior.
- The ischial tuberosity is the common attachment for the hamstrings (semimembranosus, semitendinosus, and biceps femoris).
- Note the appropriate use of a gonad shield.

Question 8:

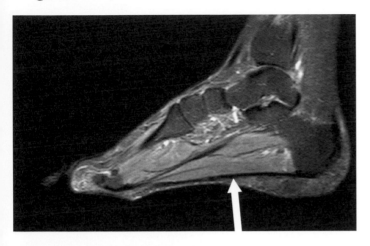

Name the arrowed structure	

Question 9:

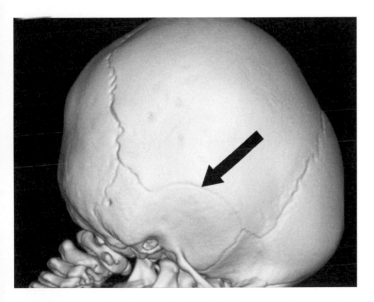

Name the arrowed structure	

▪ Question 8: Sagittal MRI of the foot

Answer: Plantar fascia

- The plantar fascia (or plantar aponeurosis) is a strong fibrous layer that connects the calcaneal tuberosity to the heads of the metatarsal bones and supports the arch of the foot.
- It is well delineated on sagittal MRI studies and appears as a uniform hypointense band at the sole of the foot.

▪ Question 9: Surface rendered 3D reconstruction of a paediatric skull

Answer: Right temporoparietal (squamosal) suture

- There are three main sutures in the skull: the sagittal suture, the paired lambdoid, and paired coronal sutures.
- Other sutures that may be visible depending on the age of the child are the temporoparietal suture, sphenotemporal suture, and metopic suture.
- The pterion is where the sphenoparietal suture joins the coronal suture.
- The asterion is where the temporoparietal suture joins the lambdoid suture.

▪ Question 10:

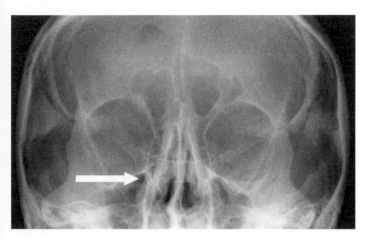

Name the arrowed structure	

■ Question 10: Orbital radiograph

Answer: Right foramen rotundum

- The foramen rotundum runs from the middle cranial fossa to the pterygopalatine fossa in the sphenoid bone.
- It transmits the maxillary division of the trigeminal nerve (V_2).
- The table below summarises the structures that pass through the skull base and various facial foramina. Questions on this area are common.

Facial/Skull Foramina	Contents
Optic canal	Optic nerve ophthalmic artery
Superior orbital fissure	Cranial nerves III, IV, ophthalmic nerve (V_1), VI Superior orbital vein, branch of middle meningeal artery
Inferior orbital fissure	Infraorbital nerve and artery, inferior ophthalmic veins
Foramen rotundum	Maxillary nerve (V_2)
Foramen ovale	Mandibular nerve (V_3), accessory meningeal artery
Foramen spinosum	Middle meningeal artery
Foramen lacerum	Internal carotid artery
Internal auditory meatus	Cranial nerves VII and VIII
Jugular foramen	Cranial nerves IX, X and XI, internal jugular vein, inferior petrosal and sigmoid sinuses
Hypoglossal canal	Cranial nerve XII

Middle cranial fossa
Posterior cranial fossa

Question 11:

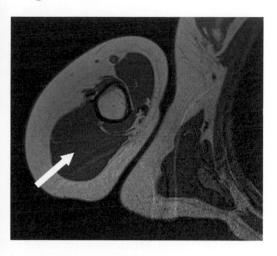

Name the arrowed structure	

Question 12:

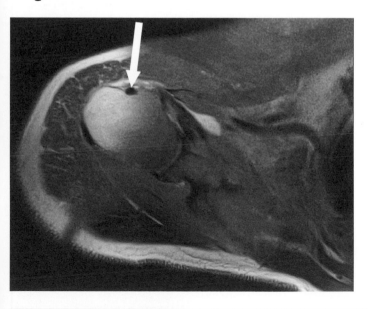

Name the arrowed structure	

▪ Question 11: Axial MRI of the upper limb

Answer: Triceps brachii muscle

• As its name infers, the triceps brachii ('three headed muscle of the arm') muscle is formed from three proximal muscle bundles (long/lateral/medial heads) that arise from the posterior aspect of the upper limb to join together at the elbow before inserting onto the olecranon process of the ulna.

▪ Question 12: Axial MRI of the shoulder

Answer: Biceps brachii muscle tendon (long head)

• As its name infers, the biceps brachii ('two headed muscle of the arm') muscle is formed by two proximal muscle bundles: the short head originating from the coracoid process of the scapula, and the long head from the supraglenoid tubercle.
• The long head has a tendon that passes within the bicipital groove (intertubercular groove) of the humerus.
• The heads join at mid humeral level to form a common muscle belly before inserting into the radial tuberosity.

Question 13:

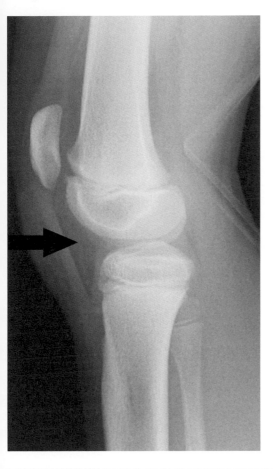

Name the arrowed structure	

▪ Question 13: Lateral radiograph of the knee

Answer: Hoffa's fat pad

- The Hoffa's fat pad is the fat pad posterior to the patellar tendon and anterior to the knee joint.
- Fat is low density so it appears dark on plain radiography. On both T1- and T2-weighted MRI sequences, fat will appear high intensity (bright).
- A fluid level in the Hoffa's fat pad or within the suprapatellar recess of the joint is called a lipohaemarthrosis and is a direct sign of an intra-articular fracture.

Question 14:

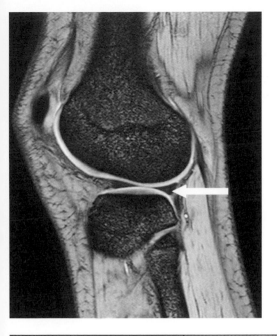

Name the arrowed structure	

▪ Question 14: T1-weighted sagittal MRI of the knee

Answer: Posterior horn of the lateral meniscus

- The menisci are best seen on sagittal or coronal MRI and appear as black triangles. Degeneration or a tear will usually appear as high (bright) signal.
- It is important that your response to this question be precise. Because the fibula is seen on this slice, you can be sure that this is the lateral meniscus. Determining which is the anterior and posterior horn should be relatively straightforward.

Question 15:

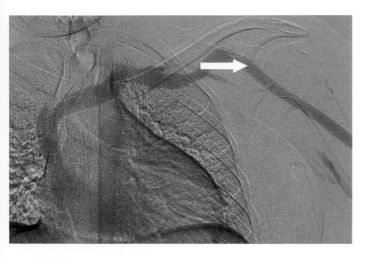

Name the arrowed structure	

Question 16:

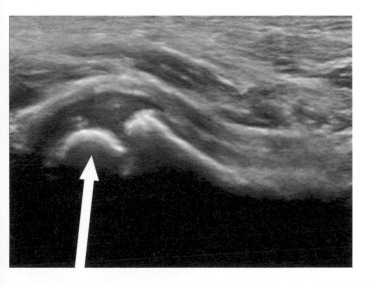

Name the arrowed structure	

■ Question 15: Upper Limb venogram

Answer: Left axillary vein

- The axillary vein forms from the confluence of the brachial, basilic, and cephalic veins.
- It becomes the subclavian vein as it passes underneath the lateral border of the first rib.
- The cephalic vein originates from the confluence of the radial aspect of the dorsal venous plexus of the hand and ascends proximally up the forearm and arm. It pierces the clavipectoral fascia and drains into the axillary vein.
- The basilic vein originates from the confluence of the ulnar aspect of the dorsal venous plexus of the hand and ascends proximally up the forearm and forms the axillary vein.
- The basilic and cephalic veins communicate at the cubital fossa via the median cubital vein.

■ Question 16: Ultrasound of an infant's hip

Answer: Femoral head

- Paediatric ultrasound images of the hip are very common in the examination.
- Be familiar with the sagittal view. Orientate yourself with the round femoral head. Visualise the Y-shaped arrangement of the ilium/labrum/acetabular roof, which forms a caplike structure on the femoral head.
- The iliopsoas muscle can be seen as the superficial structure along the axis of imaging.

■ **Question 17:**

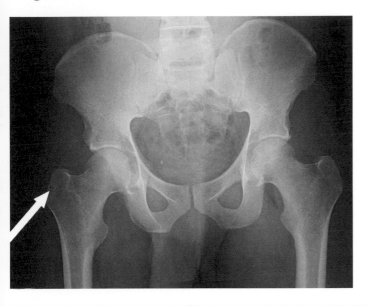

What muscle attaches here?	

■ Question 17: AP radiograph of the pelvis

Answer: Right gluteus medius muscle

- The gluteus medius muscle attaches to the lateral aspect of the greater trochanter.
- The obturator externus and the superior and inferior gemellus muscles attach to the medial aspect of the greater trochanter.

Question 18:

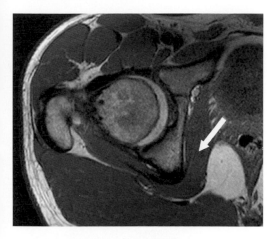

Name the arrowed structure	

▪ Question 18: Axial MRI of the right hip

Answer: Right obturator internus muscle

- The obturator internus muscle originates from the obturator membrane.
- It traverses the lesser sciatic foramen and inserts onto the greater trochanter of the femur.

■ Question 19:

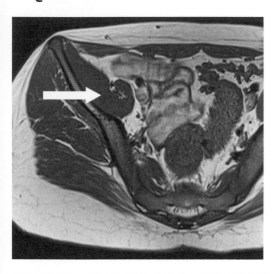

Name the arrowed structure	

■ Question 20:

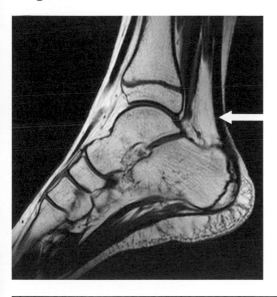

Name the arrowed structure	

■ Question 19: T1-weighted axial MRI of the pelvis

Answer: Right iliacus muscle

- The iliacus muscle sits in the inner aspect of the iliac bone, lateral to the inferior part of psoas major.
- It attaches to the superior two thirds of the iliac fossa and joins the psoas tendon to form the iliopsoas, which inserts onto the lesser trochanter of the femur. It is innervated by the femoral nerve.
- Its function is to flex the thigh and stabilise the hip joint.

■ Question 20: T1-weighted sagittal MRI of the ankle

Answer: Achilles tendon

- The Achilles tendon is the conjoined tendon of the gastrocnemius and soleus muscles.
- The musculotendinous junction is approximately 6 cm proximal to the insertion onto the posterior aspect of the calcaneum.
- On MRI, it appears as a low intensity (black) structure on T1-weighted and proton density sequences. On US, it appears as a thin (approximately 6 mm) reflective fibrous structure.
- Note the unfused distal tibial epiphysis, which indicates that this is a young patient.

▪ Question 21:

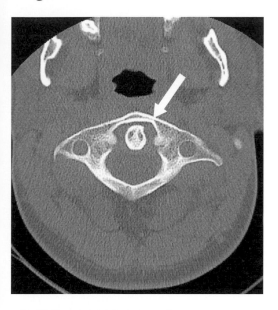

Name the arrowed structure	

▪ Question 22:

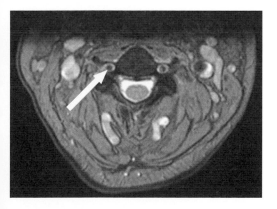

Name the arrowed structure	

■ Question 21: Axial CT of the neck

Answer: Anterior arch of the atlas (C1)

- Unlike other vertebrae, the atlas does not have a body. It is shaped like a ring with lateral masses on either side.
- Each lateral mass has superior and inferior facets for articulation with the occiput at the atlanto-occipital joint and axis (C2) at the atlantoaxial joint.
- The anterior arch has a tubercle on the anterior surface and a posterior facet that articulates with the odontoid process.
- A pair of vertebral arteries exit from the foramen transversarium and form grooves on the posterior arch as it passes alongside the lateral masses before entering the foramen magnum.

■ Question 22: T2-weighted axial MRI of the neck

Answer: Right vertebral artery

- The vertebral arteries originate from the subclavian arteries and ascend through the foramen transversarium from the level of C6.
- They enter the foramen magnum and join at the base of the medulla oblongata to form the basilar artery.

Question 23:

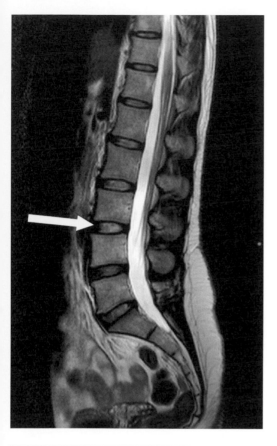

Name the arrowed structure	

■ Question 23: T2-weighted sagittal MRI of the spine

Answer: L3/4 intervertebral disc

- Intervertebral discs form fibrocartilaginous joints between successive vertebral bodies.
- They are amphiarthrodial joints (meaning that limited movement is possible) and, in effect, act as a ligament to maintain vertebral alignment.
- The intervertebral discs constitute one fifth of the vertebral column height.
- Intervertebral discs are wedge-shaped in the cervical and lumbar regions, contributing to spine lordosis. The thoracic intervertebral discs are rectangular in shape.
- Each intervertebral disc is composed of an outer annulus fibrosus, a central nucleus pulposus, and cartilaginous endplates.

▪ Question 24:

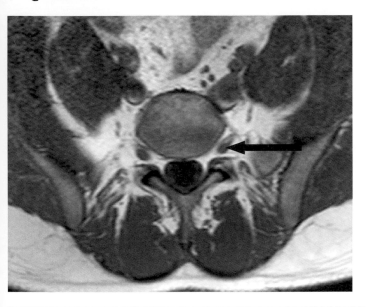

Name the arrowed structure	

▪ Question 25:

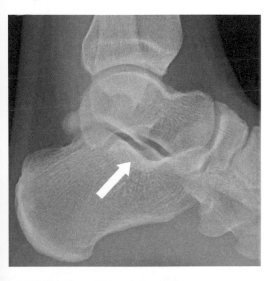

Name the arrowed structure	

■ Question 24: Axial MRI of the lumbar spine

Answer: Left spinal nerve root (exiting nerve root)

- There are 31 segmental nerve roots that arise from each side of the spinal cord: 8 cervical, 12 thoracic, 5 lumbar, 5 sacral, and 1 coccygeal.
- Each spinal nerve root is formed by the union of a dorsal root (sensory) and a ventral root (motor and autonomic). It passes anterolaterally through the neural/intervertebral foramen before dividing into ventral and dorsal rami.
- Spinal nerve roots of C1-C7 exit above the pedicles of their respective vertebrae. Because there is no C8 vertebra, subsequent nerve roots exit below the pedicles of their respective vertebrae.

■ Question 25: Lateral radiograph of the ankle

Answer: Sustentaculum tali

- The calcaneus is a complex bone. It articulates anteriorly with the cuboid and cranially with the talus.
- The sustentaculum tali, also known as the talar shelf, is a horizontal eminence on the medial aspect of the calcaneus that serves as the site of ligamentous attachment.

▪ Question 26:

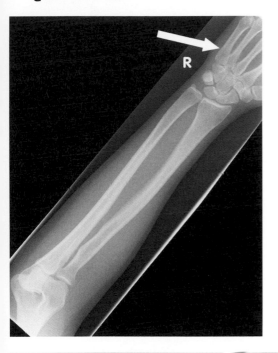

Name the arrowed structure	

▪ Question 26: AP radiograph of the forearm

Answer: Right little finger metacarpal

• Each metacarpal bone can be divided into three parts: head, body, and base.

▪ Question 27:

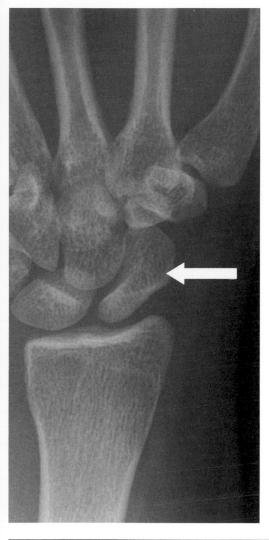

Name the arrowed structure	

■ Question 27: Plain radiograph of the wrist

Answer: Scaphoid bone

- The scaphoid bone has a boatlike configuration and can be divided into the proximal pole and distal pole with the waist in between.
- It is the largest of the proximal carpal row bones.
- It articulates proximally with the radius, lunate, capitate, trapezoid, and trapezium.
- It is perfused in a retrograde fashion by a single branch from the radial artery.

▪ Question 28:

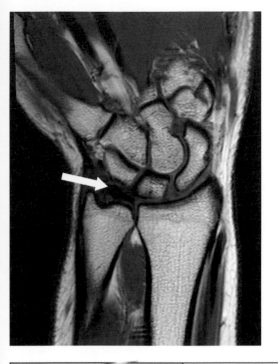

Name the arrowed structure	

▪ Question 28: Coronal MRI of the wrist

Answer: Triangular fibrocartilaginous complex

- As the name suggests, the triangular fibrocartilaginous complex is composed of a fibrocartilaginous articular disc with ligaments that originate from the medial border of the distal radius and inserts into the ulna styloid.
- It is triangular in shape and serves as the main stabilizer of the distal radioulnar joint and supports the distal carpal row.

Question 29:

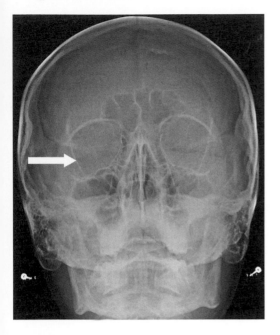

Name the arrowed structure	

▪ Question 29: Frontal radiograph of the facial bones

Answer: Greater wing of the right sphenoid bone (innominate line)

- There are many different facial and temporal bones; they can be difficult to remember.
- The sphenoid bone consists of a body, greater and lesser wings, and forms part of the skull base.
- The greater wing appears as a high density line due to the tangential projection.

■ Question 30:

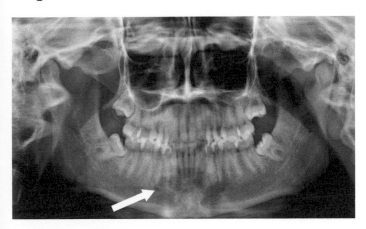

Name the arrowed structure	

■ Question 31:

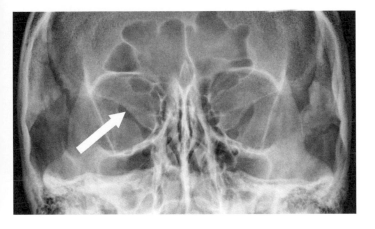

Name the arrowed structure	

▪ Question 30: Orthopantomogram

Answer: Right mental foramen

- The mental foramina are best seen, but are not always visible, on the orthopantomogram.
- The orthopantomogram is a panoramic projection that converts a curved 3D structure into a 2D image.
- The mental foramina are seen as small, round, transradiant structures because each contains fat and the mental nerve, not bone.
- They lie inferior to the roots of the teeth and lateral to the mental symphysis.

▪ Question 31: Orbital radiograph

Answer: Right superior orbital fissure

- The superior orbital fissure contains cranial nerves III, IV, V_1, and VI; superior orbital vein; and a branch of the middle meningeal artery.
- It is a triangular space between the greater and lesser wings of the sphenoid.

▪ Question 32:

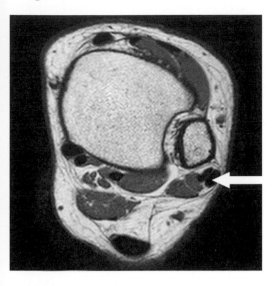

Name the arrowed structure	

▪ Question 32: T1-weighted axial MRI of the ankle

Answer: Left peroneus longus tendon

- There are two principal peroneus tendons: longus and brevis. There are several accessory peroneus tendons (e.g. peroneus tertius).
- They both run a lateral course posterior to the lateral malleolus.
- Peroneus longus is lateral to peroneus brevis.
- It runs inferior to the cuboid bone, crosses the foot, and inserts onto the base of the first metatarsal and medial cuneiform.
- Peroneus brevis inserts onto the base of the fifth metatarsal.

Question 33:

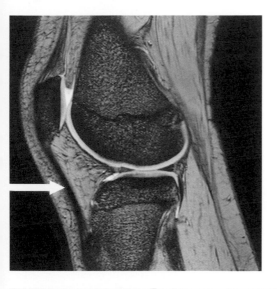

Name the arrowed structure	

Question 34:

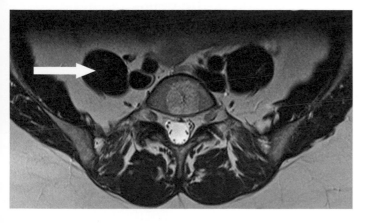

Name the arrowed structure	

■ Question 33: Sagittal T2-weighted MRI of the knee

Answer: Patellar tendon

- On US, the patellar tendon appears as a slightly hyperreflective fibrous structure. On T1-weighted/proton density MRI, it is a low intensity (black) band.
- It runs from the patella to the tibial tuberosity.

■ Question 34: T2-weighted axial MRI of the pelvis

Answer: Right psoas major muscle

- The paired psoas major muscles run laterally from the lumbar vertebrae.
- They attach superiorly to the transverse processes of T12-L5 and the lumbar vertebral bodies.
- Psoas major joins the iliacus muscle to form the iliopsoas, which inserts onto the lesser trochanter of the femur.
- *Psoas* is Greek for 'loin'. A beef tenderloin or fillet is actually the psoas muscle.

Question 35:

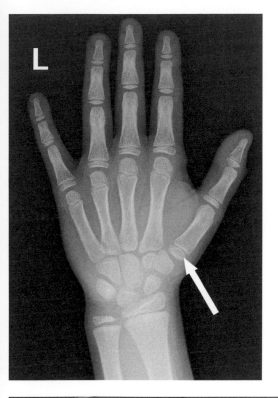

Name the arrowed structure	

▪ Question 35: AP radiograph of the left hand

Answer: Epiphysis of the left thumb metacarpal

- The epiphysis of the thumb metacarpal is at the base of the metacarpal diaphysis.
- This differs from the epiphyses of the other metacarpals, where it is situated distal to the metacarpal diaphysis.

Question 36:

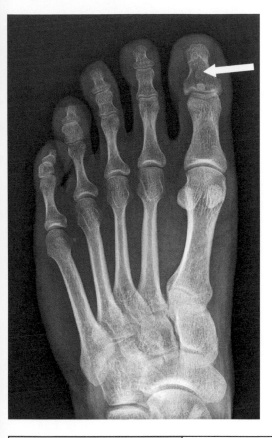

Name the arrowed structure	

■ Question 36: AP radiograph of the left foot

Answer: Distal phalanx of the left great toe

- The flexor hallucis longus muscle is the most powerful muscle within the posterior compartment of the leg—the other muscles being flexor digitorum longus and tibialis posterior.
- The flexor hallucis longus muscle originates from the middle third of the fibula and travels in an oblique direction down the leg and under the sustentaculum tali of the calcaneus to run on the plantar aspect of the foot and inserts into the base of the great toe distal phalanx.

▪ Question 37:

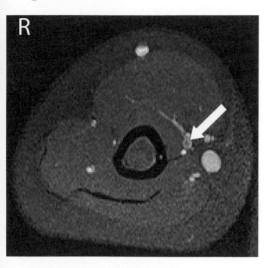

Name the arrowed structure	

▪ Question 37: Axial MRI of the right arm

Answer: Right brachial artery

- Although detailed knowledge of neurovascular anatomy is not required for the examination, do not neglect it as part of your revision because it is a common topic.
- The brachial artery is the distal continuation of the axillary artery beyond the lower margin of teres minor muscle. It bifurcates into the radial and ulnar arteries, which run through the forearm.
- At the elbow joint, the biceps brachii tendon lies lateral to the brachial artery.

■ Question 38:

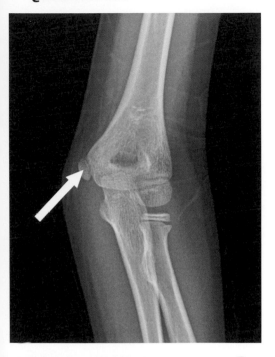

Name the arrowed structure	

■ Question 38: AP radiograph of the left elbow

Answer: Ossification centre of the left internal (medial) epicondyle

- Knowing when the different ossification centres appear is essential for this question.
- The acronym CRITOL can be used:

C	Capitulum (or capitellum)	1 year
R	Radial head	3 years
I	Internal epicondyle	5 years
T	Trochlear	10 years
O	Olecranon	10 years
L	Lateral epicondyle	11 years

■ Question 39:

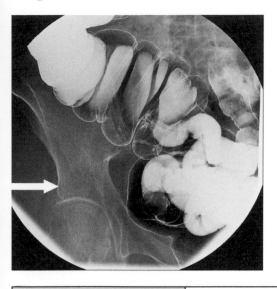

Name the arrowed structure	

■ Question 39: Barium enema

Answer: Right anterior inferior iliac spine

- The anterior inferior iliac spine is the attachment for the rectus femoris muscle.
- The barium within the colon is there to act as a distraction from what is actually a simple question to answer.
- The table below summarises the main sites of muscle attachment in the pelvis and the corresponding muscles that insert there.

Pelvic attachment	Muscle(s)
Iliac crest	Abdominal wall muscles (external oblique, internal oblique, and transversus abdominis)
Anterior superior iliac spine	Sartorius
Anterior inferior iliac spine	Rectus femoris
Inferior pubic ramus	Adductors (adductor longus, brevis, and magnus; and gracilis)
Ischial tuberosity	Hamstrings (semimembranosus, semitendinosus, and biceps femoris)
Greater trochanter	Gluteus medius
Lesser trochanter	Iliopsoas

▪ Question 40:

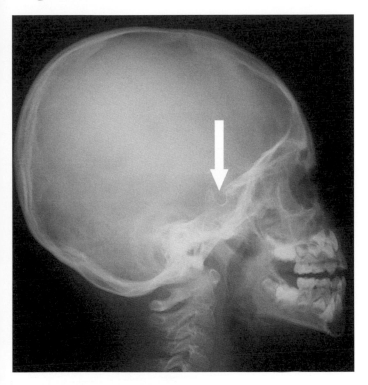

Name the arrowed structure	

■ Question 40: Lateral skull radiograph

Answer: Sella turcica or pituitary fossa

- The sella turcica is a deep fossa within the sphenoid bone that contains the pituitary gland.
- The anterior part of the sella turcica is the tuberculum sellae, and the posterior part is the dorsum sellae. The clinoid processes—two posterior and two anterior—are bony projections that surround the sella turcica.

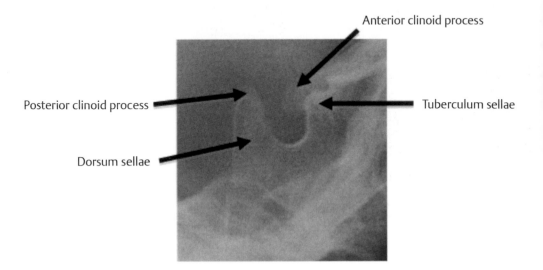

Question 41:

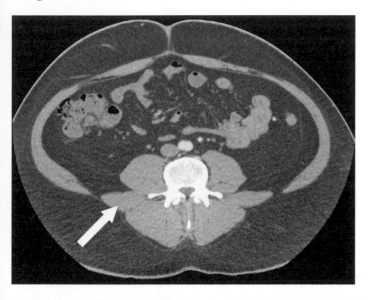

Name the arrowed structure	

■ Question 41: Axial contrast-enhanced CT of the abdomen

Answer: Right quadratus lumborum muscle

- The quadratus lumborum muscle is one of the muscles of the posterior abdominal wall. The others are psoas major, iliacus, external oblique, internal oblique, and transversus abdominis.
- It is quadrilateral in shape.
- It lies lateral to the lumbar transverse processes, posterior to the psoas major, and anterior to erector spinae.
- Lateral to quadratus lumborum is the lumbar triangle, a potential site of abdominal herniation.

Question 42:

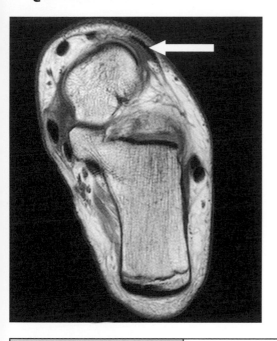

Name the arrowed structure	

▪ Question 42: Axial oblique MRI of the ankle

Answer: Extensor digitorum longus

- There are four muscles in the anterior compartment of the lower leg: tibialis anterior, extensor digitorum longus, extensor hallucis longus, and peroneus tertius.
- Extensor digitorum longus extends from the lateral condyle of the tibia to insert on the middle and distal phalanges of the second to fifth toes.
- It dorsiflexes the ankle.

Question 43:

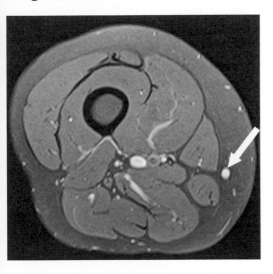

Name the arrowed structure	

▪ Question 43: Axial MRI of the upper thigh

Answer: Great (long) saphenous vein

- The great saphenous vein is a superficial vein formed from the dorsal venous arch and dorsal vein of the great toe.
- It runs medially from anterior to the medial malleolus up the length of the leg to drain into the femoral vein in the inguinal region.
- Communicating veins connect the saphenous vein to the deep veins.
- The short saphenous vein is on the lateral aspect of the lower leg and drains into the popliteal vein.
- Because the great saphenous vein is a medial structure, you can be sure that this is the right leg and thus right great saphenous vein.

▪ Question 44:

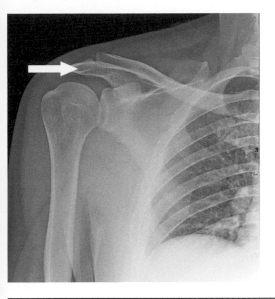

Name the arrowed structure	

■ Question 44: Plain radiograph of the right shoulder

Answer: Right acromion process

- The acromion is the superolateral continuation of the scapular spine.
- It is triangular in configuration and bends anterolaterally to form the summit of the shoulder.
- It articulates with the clavicle at the acromioclavicular joint.
- The acromion has four ossification centres, which usually fuse by adulthood. Failure of one of the ossification centres to fuse will result in an os acromiale.

▪ Question 45:

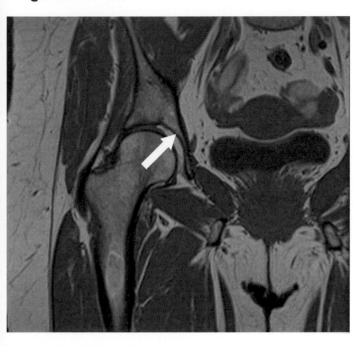

Name the arrowed structure	

▪ Question 45: T1-weighted coronal MRI of the pelvis

Answer: Right acetabulum

- The hip bones (ilium, ischium, and pubis) unite to form the acetabulum.
- It has a smooth concave surface and is marked by a depression in its inferior portion called the acetabular notch.
- It is covered by a C-shaped layer of fibrocartilaginous labrum, which deepens the acetabulum and increases articular surface area with the femoral head.

Question 46:

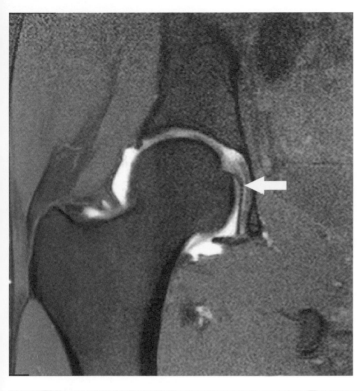

Name the arrowed structure	

▪ Question 46: Coronal MRI arthrogram of the right hip

Answer: Right ligamentum teres femoris (ligament of the head of the femur)

- The ligamentum teres femoris is a flat band that spans across the hip joint from acetabular notch to the fovea capitis femoris.
- It contains the acetabular branch of the medial circumflex femoral artery.
- Please distinguish between the ligamentum teres femoris from the ligamentum teres uteri and the ligamentum teres hepatis.

Question 47:

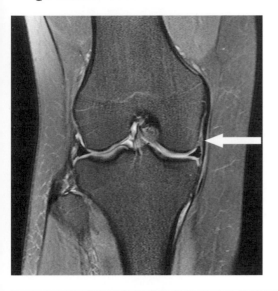

Name the arrowed structure	

Question 48:

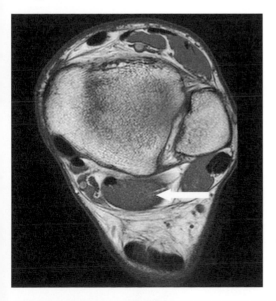

Name the arrowed structure	

▪ Question 47: Coronal proton density MRI of the knee

Answer: Medial collateral ligament

- The medial collateral ligament (MCL) can be seen as a complete structure on one slice unlike the lateral collateral ligament, which is seen on two or three slices.
- The MCL appears as a uniform low intensity (black) structure.
- It originates from the medial femoral epicondyle and inserts onto the medial tibial condyle.
- The MCL is firmly attached to the medial meniscus, which is why injuries to these structures often occur together.

▪ Question 48: T1-weighted axial MRI of the ankle

Answer: Left flexor hallucis longus muscle

- There are three main flexor tendons found in the posterior lower leg: tibialis posterior, flexor digitorum longus, and flexor hallucis longus. This can be remembered by 'Tom, Dick, and Harry' (from medial to lateral).
- For the extensor tendons, it is Tom (tibialis anterior), Harry (extensor hallucis longus), and Dick (extensor digitorum longus) from medial to lateral.
- Flexor hallucis longus attaches to the base of the distal phalanx of the great toe.
- If the arrow is clearly pointing to the muscle belly (grey) or the tendon (black), then it is better to be precise in your answer. If you are unsure, you could leave off the muscle or tendon part of the answer.

Question 49:

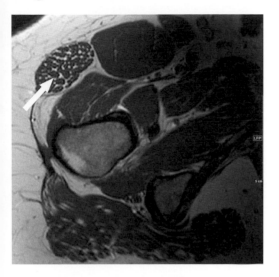

Name the arrowed structure	

■ Question 49: T1-weighted axial MRI of the right hip

Answer: Right tensor fasciae latae

- The tensor fasciae latae is a muscle found on the lateral aspect of the thigh. It originates from the iliac crest and inserts into the iliotibial tract.
- It is characterised by patchy fatty areas on axial imaging; thus, look for areas of low attenuation on CT and high signal on T1- and T2-weighted MRI.

Question 50:

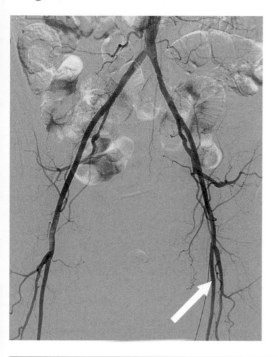

Name the arrowed structure	

▪ Question 50: Iliac angiogram

Answer: Left superficial femoral artery

- Although detailed knowledge of vascular anatomy is not required for the examination, do not neglect it as part of your revision because it is a common topic.
- The external iliac artery continues below the level of the inguinal ligament as the common femoral artery, which bifurcates into the superficial femoral artery and deep femoral artery.
- The superficial femoral artery passes inferomedially and emerges as the popliteal artery after exiting the Hunter's canal (adductor canal).

Chapter 5

Mock Examination

Question 1:

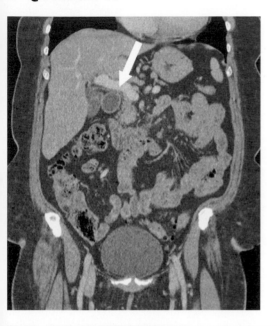

Name the arrowed structure	

▪ Question 2:

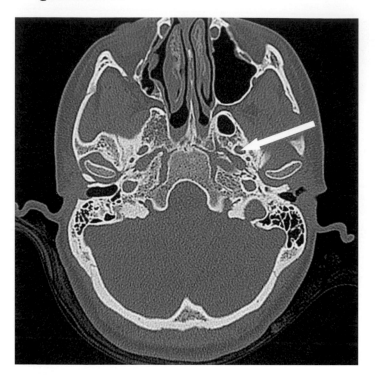

Which nerves pass through this structure?	

▪ Question 3:

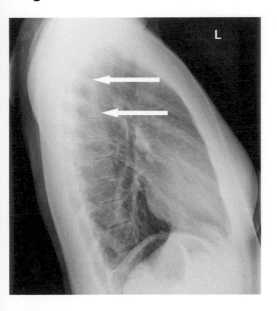

Name the arrowed structure	

▪ Question 4:

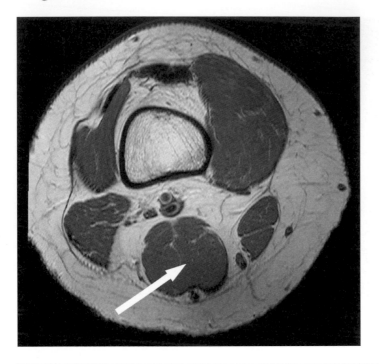

Name the arrowed structure	

Question 5:

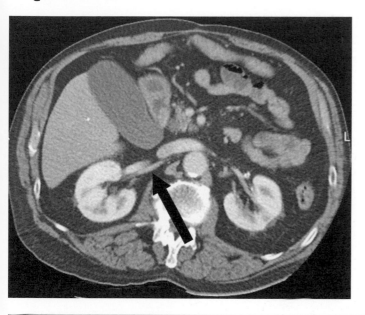

Name the arrowed structure	

Question 6:

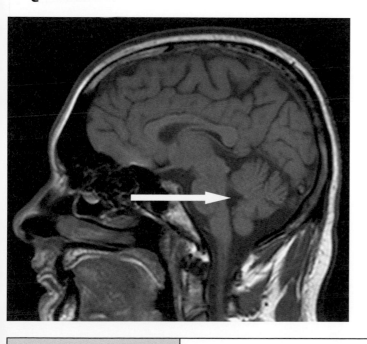

Name the arrowed structure	

Question 7:

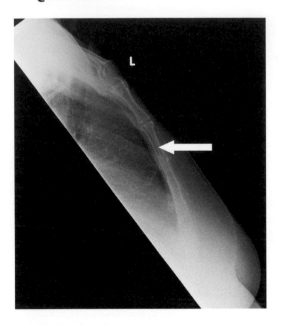

Name the arrowed structure	

▪ Question 8:

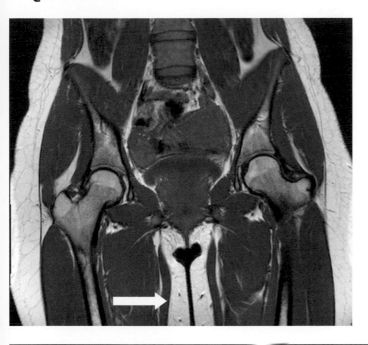

Name the arrowed structure	

Question 9:

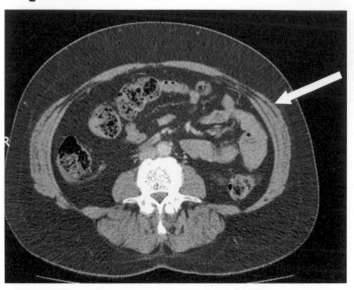

Name the arrowed structure	

Question 10:

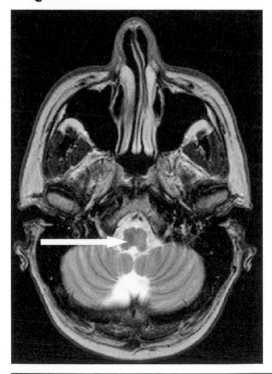

Name the arrowed structure	

Question 11:

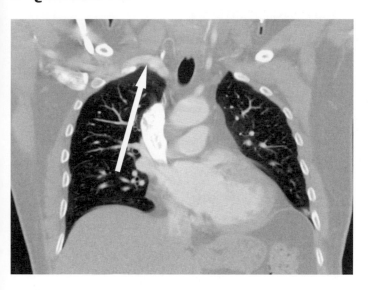

Name the arrowed structure	

Question 12:

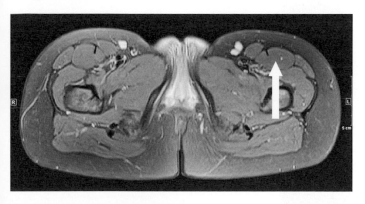

Name the arrowed structure	

▪ Question 13:

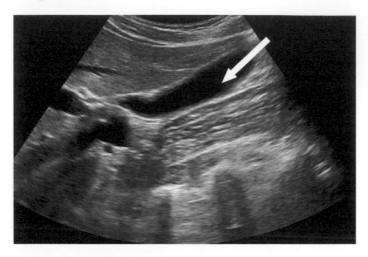

Name the arrowed structure	

▪ Question 14:

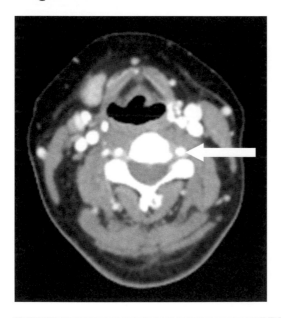

Name the arrowed structure	

Question 15:

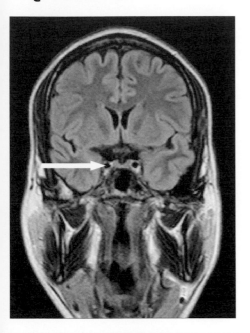

Name the arrowed structure	

■ Question 16:

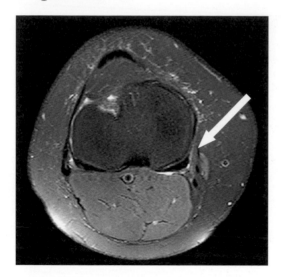

Name the arrowed structure	

Question 17:

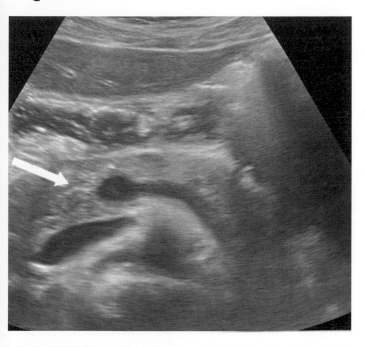

Name the arrowed structure	

Question 18:

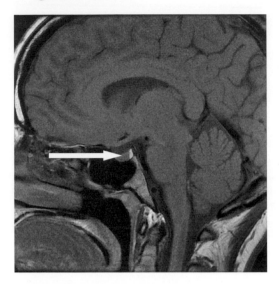

Name the arrowed structure	

Question 19:

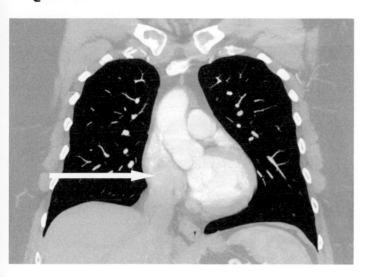

Name the arrowed structure	

Question 20:

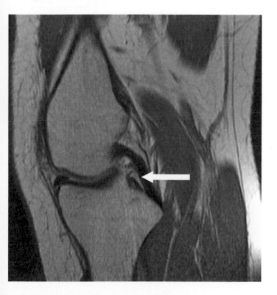

Name the arrowed structure	

- ## Question 21:

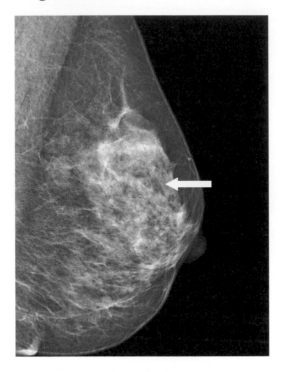

Name the arrowed structure	

Question 22:

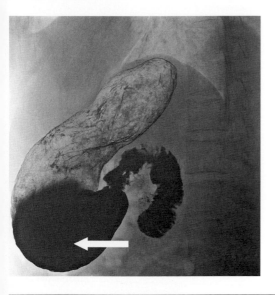

Name the arrowed structure	

■ Question 23:

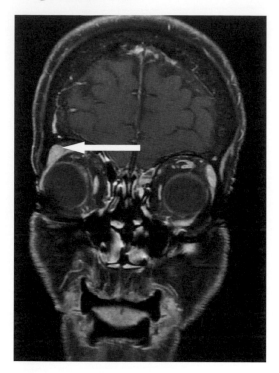

Name the arrowed structure	

▪ Question 24:

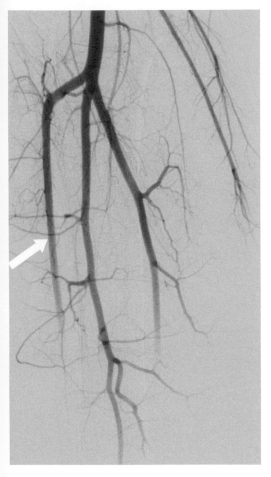

Name the arrowed structure	

▪ Question 25:

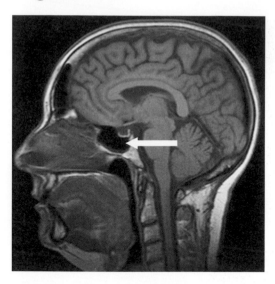

Name the arrowed structure	

Question 26:

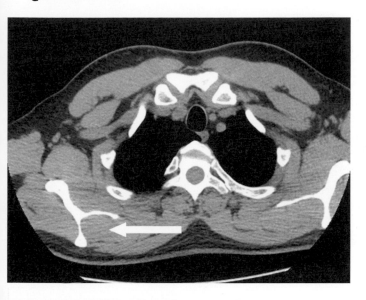

Name the arrowed structure	

Question 27:

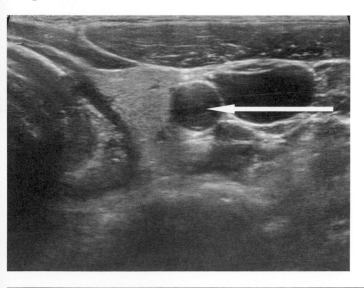

Name the arrowed structure	

■ Question 28:

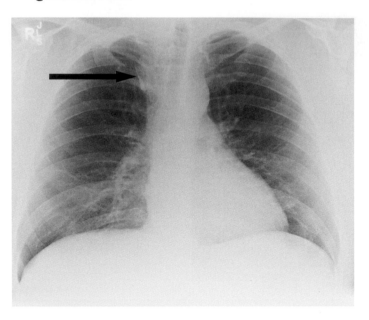

Name the arrowed structure	

■ Question 29:

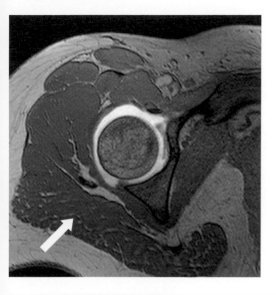

Name the arrowed structure	

▪ Question 30:

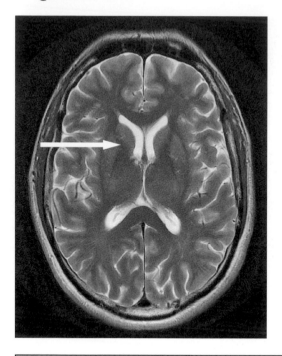

Name the arrowed structure	

■ Question 31:

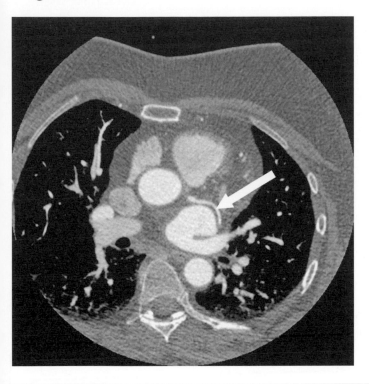

Name the arrowed structure	

■ Question 32:

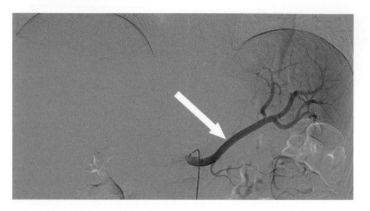

Name the arrowed structure	

■ Question 33:

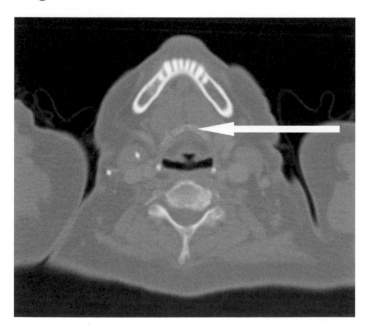

Name the arrowed structure	

Question 34:

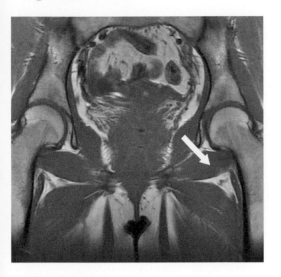

Name the arrowed structure	

Question 35:

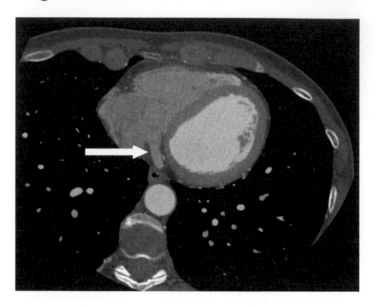

Name the arrowed structure	

Question 36:

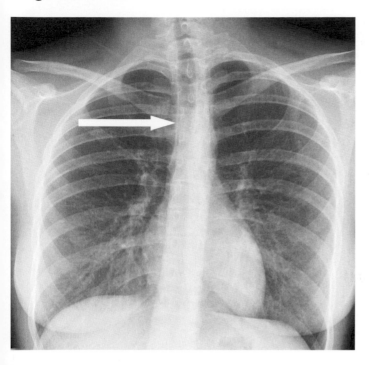

Name the arrowed structure	

■ Question 37:

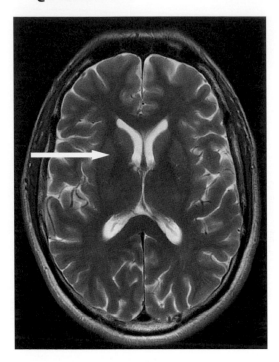

Name the arrowed structure	

▪ Question 38:

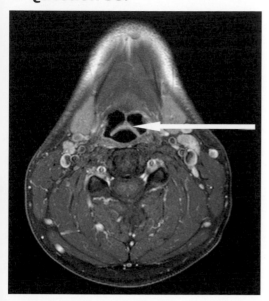

Name the arrowed structure	

▪ Question 39:

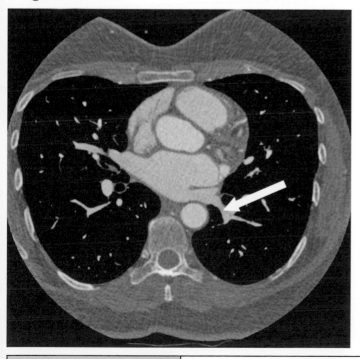

Name the arrowed structure	

Question 40:

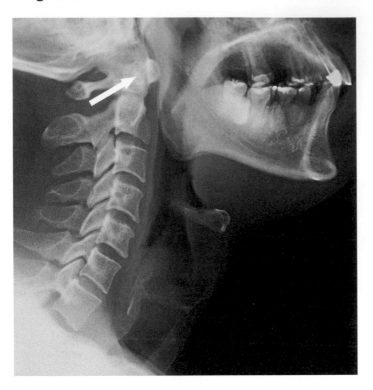

Name the arrowed structure	

Question 41:

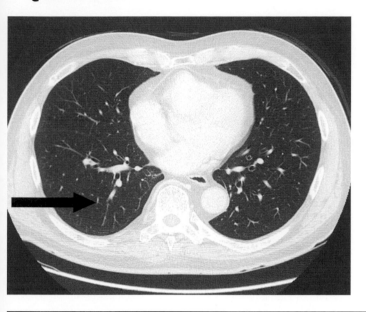

Name the arrowed structure	

- ## Question 42:

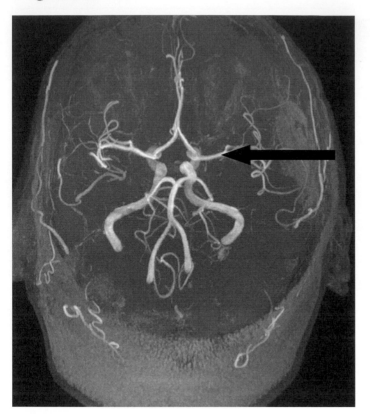

Name the arrowed structure	

Question 43:

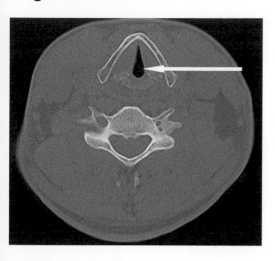

Name the arrowed structure	

Question 44:

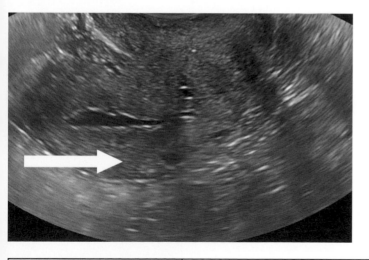

Name the arrowed structure	

- ## Question 45:

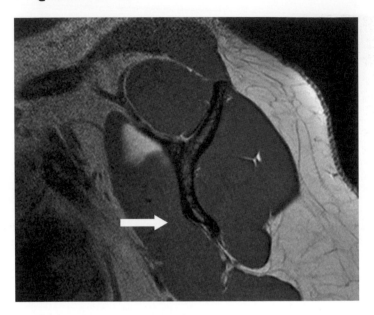

Name the arrowed structure	

Question 46:

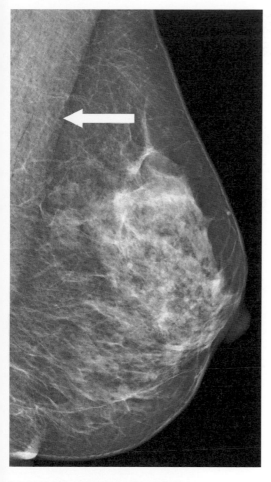

Name the arrowed structure	

■ Question 47:

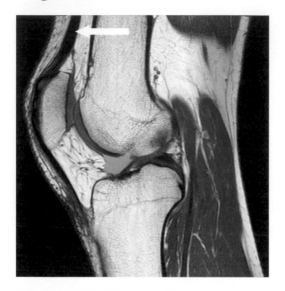

Name the arrowed structure	

Question 48:

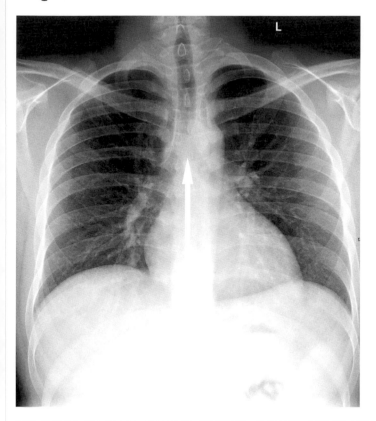

Name the arrowed structure	

■ Question 51:

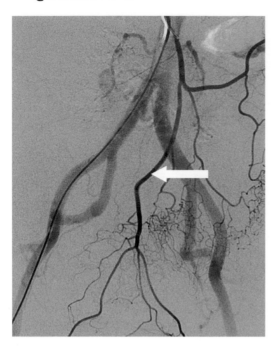

Name the arrowed structure	

Question 52:

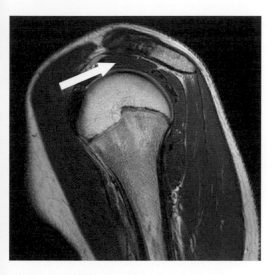

Name the arrowed structure	

▪ Question 53:

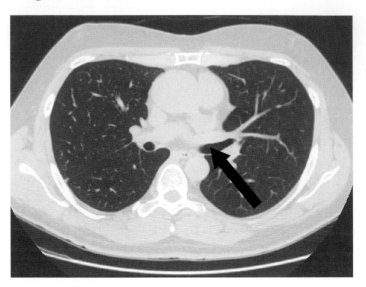

Name the arrowed structure	

Question 54:

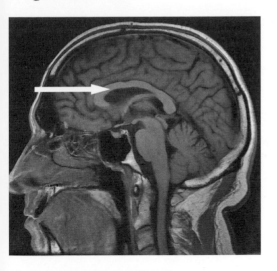

Name the arrowed structure	

■ Question 55:

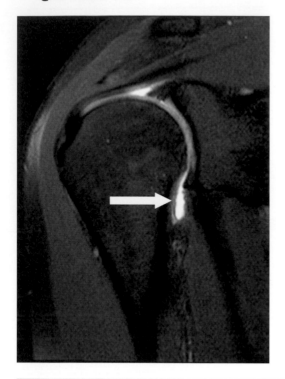

Name the arrowed structure	

Question 56:

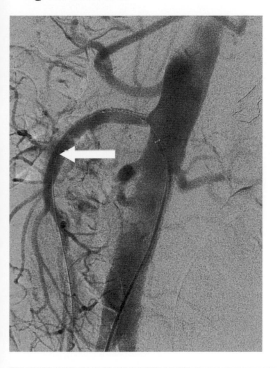

Name the arrowed structure	

- ## Question 57:

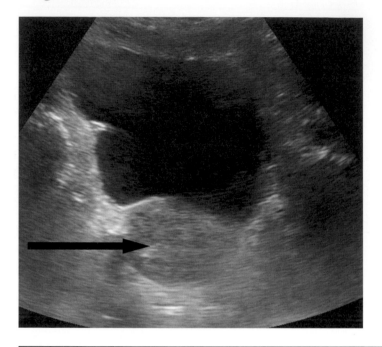

Name the arrowed structure	

- ## Question 58:

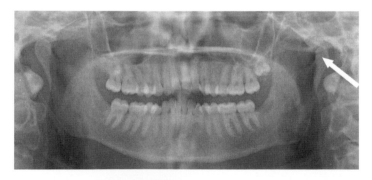

Name the arrowed structure	

Question 59:

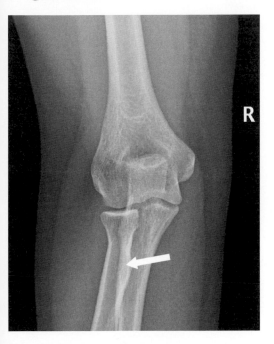

Name the arrowed structure	

Question 60:

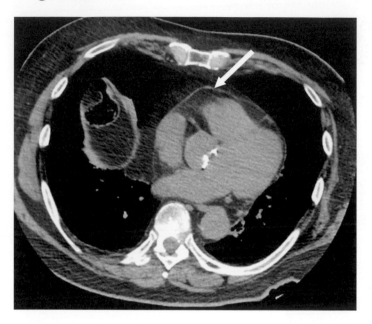

Name the arrowed structure	

■ Question 61:

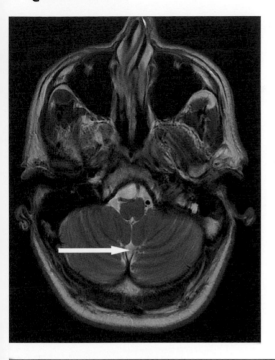

Name the arrowed structure	

■ Question 62:

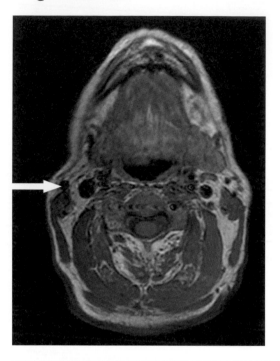

Name the arrowed structure	

Question 63:

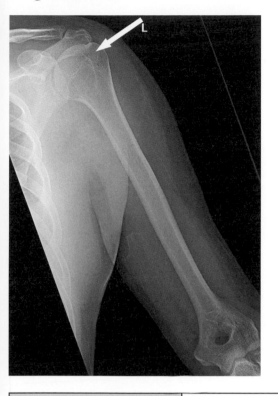

Name the arrowed structure	

■ Question 64:

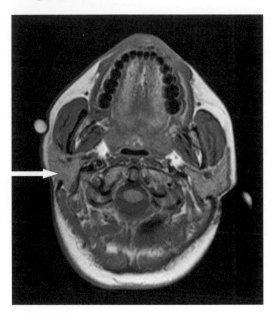

Name the arrowed structure	

▪ Question 65:

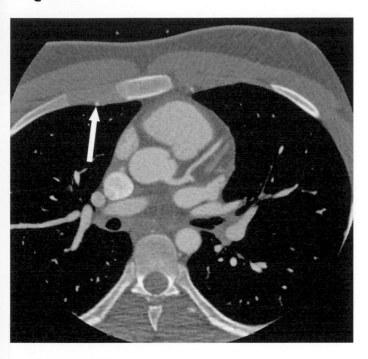

Name the arrowed structure	

■ Question 66:

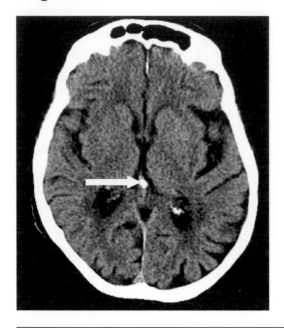

Name the arrowed structure	

■ Question 67:

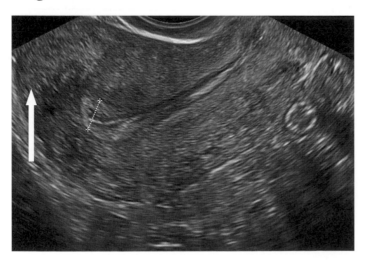

Name the arrowed structure	

Question 68:

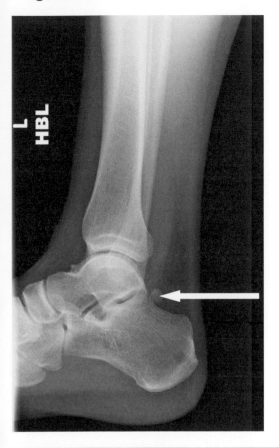

Name the arrowed structure	

▪ Question 69:

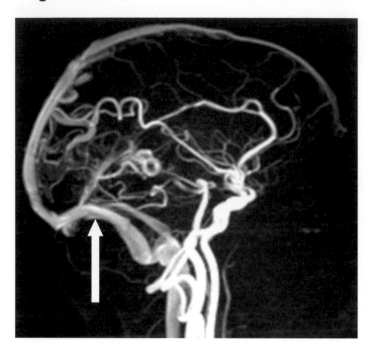

Name the arrowed structure	

Question 70:

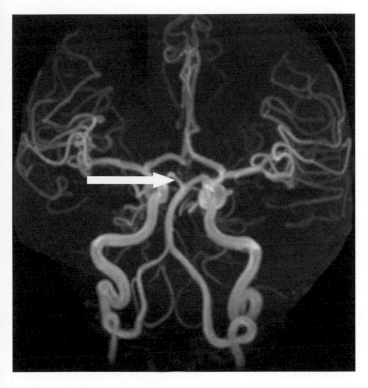

Name the arrowed structure	

■ Question 71:

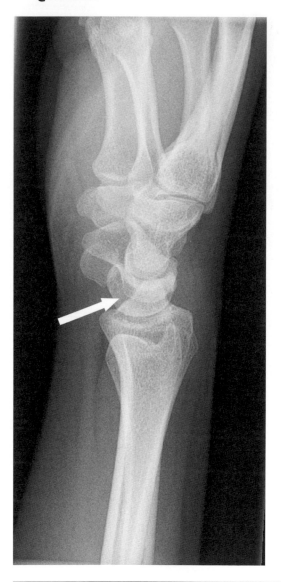

Name the arrowed structure	

Question 72:

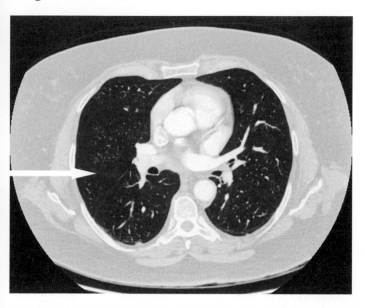

Name the arrowed structure	

▪ Question 73:

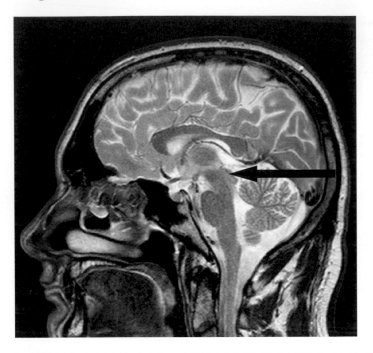

Name the arrowed structure	

Question 74:

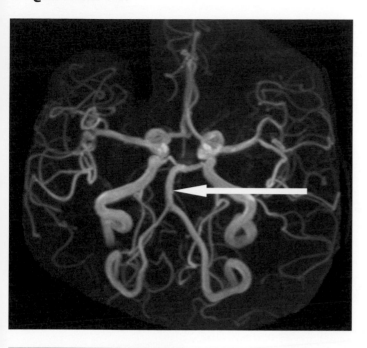

Name the arrowed structure	

▪ Question 75:

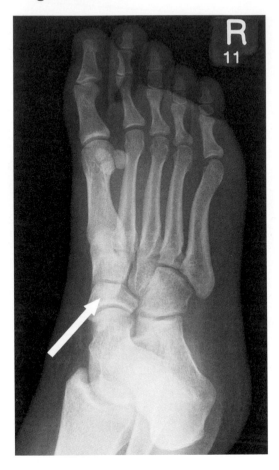

Name the arrowed structure	

▪ Question 76:

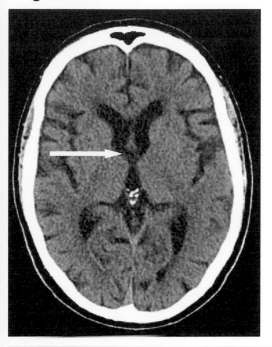

Name the arrowed structure	

▪ Question 77:

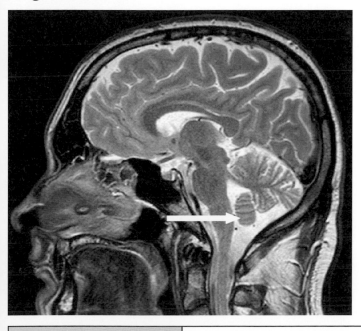

Name the arrowed structure	

▪ Question 78:

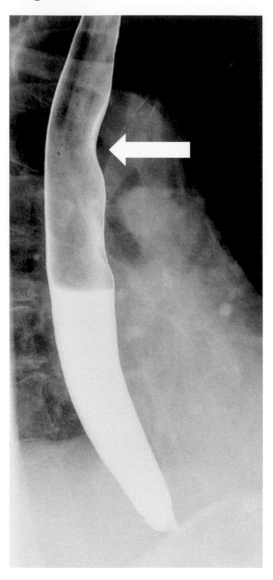

What structure causes this indentation?	

Question 79:

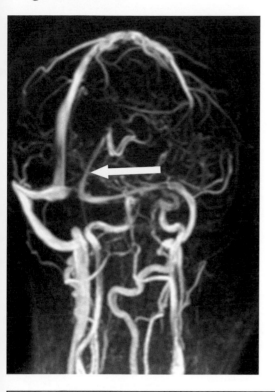

Name the arrowed structure	

■ Question 80:

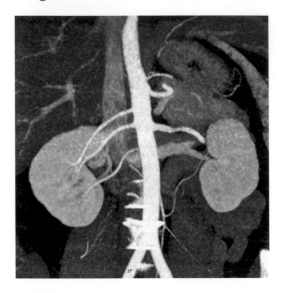

Identify the normal variant	

Question 81:

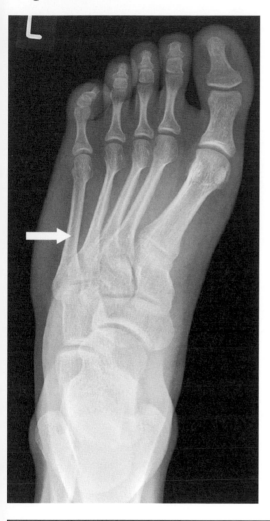

Name the arrowed structure	

- ## Question 82:

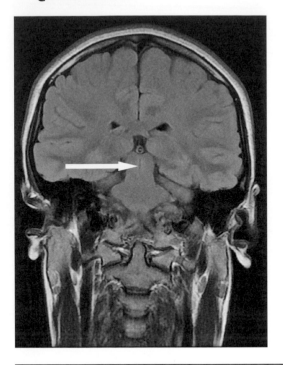

Name the arrowed structure	

Question 83:

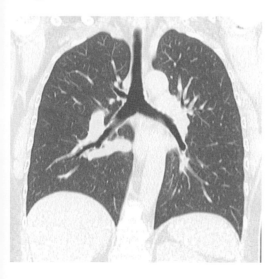

Identify the normal variant	

Question 84:

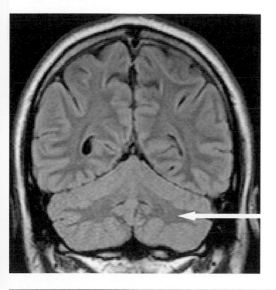

Name the arrowed structure	

▪ Question 85:

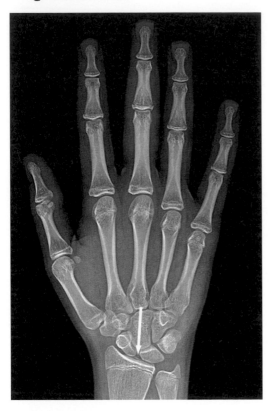

Name the arrowed structure	

▪ Question 86:

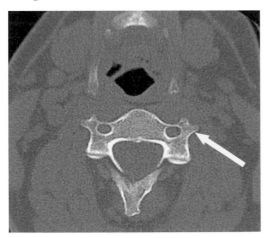

Name the arrowed structure	

Question 87:

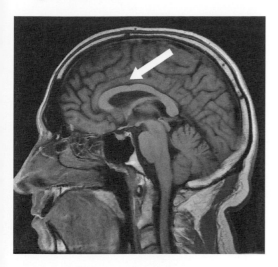

Name the arrowed structure	

Question 88:

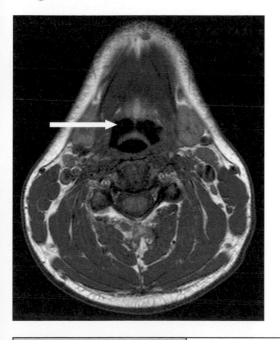

Name the arrowed structure	

■ Question 89:

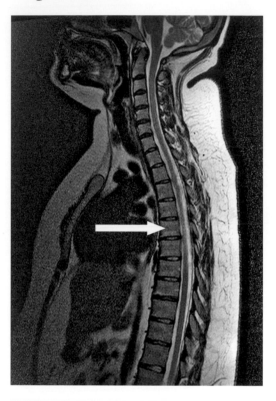

Name the arrowed structure	

▪ Question 90:

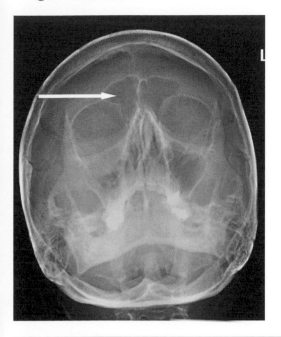

Name the arrowed structure	

▪ Question 91:

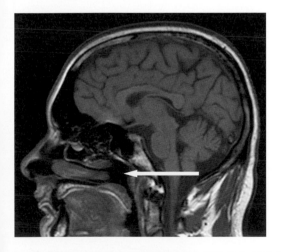

Name the arrowed structure	

▪ Question 92:

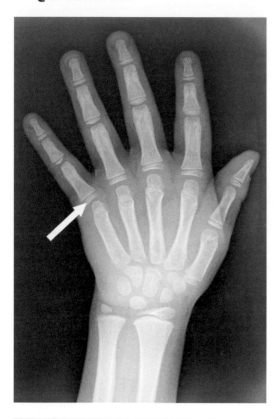

Name the arrowed structure	

Question 93:

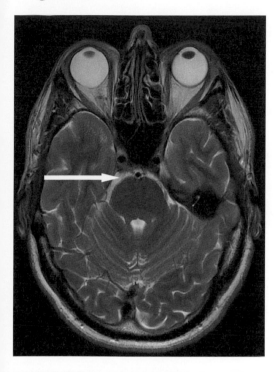

Name the arrowed structure	

▪ Question 94:

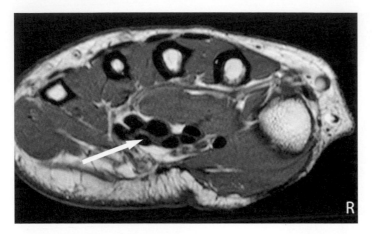

Name the arrowed structure	

Question 95:

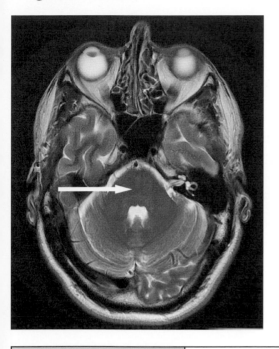

Name the arrowed structure	

Question 96:

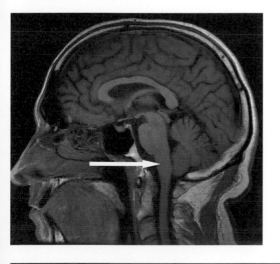

Name the arrowed structure	

■ **Question 97:**

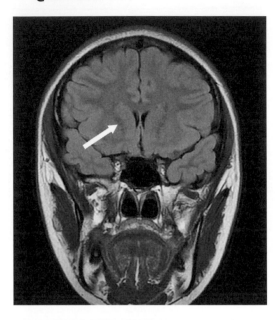

Name the arrowed structure	

Question 98:

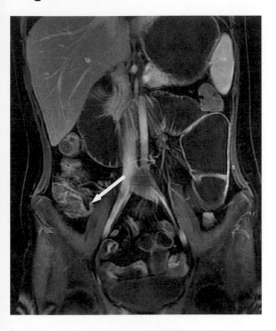

Name the arrowed structure	

■ Question 99:

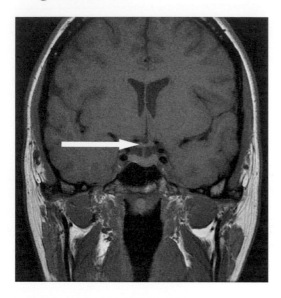

Name the arrowed structure	

Question 100:

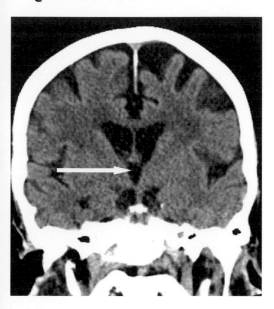

Name the arrowed structure	

ANSWERS

▪ Question 1: Coronal CT of the abdomen and pelvis

Answer: Portal vein

- The portal vein begins at the confluence of the splenic vein and superior mesenteric vein.
- The normal size of the portal vein is < 13 mm in diameter.
- Its origin defines the neck of the pancreas.

▪ Question 2: Axial CT of the petrous bones

Answer: The V_3 of the left trigeminal nerve and the left lesser petrosal nerve

- The foramen ovale is one of the larger foramina of the skull base.
- It is situated in the posterior part of the sphenoid bone.

▪ Question 3: Lateral chest radiograph

Answer: Anterior margin of scapula

- The scapula is a triangular and somewhat concave bone that occupies the posterior superolateral aspect of the thorax.
- The anterior (costal) surface is dominated by the subscapular fossa, whereas the posterior surface is divided by the scapular spine into a supraspinous fossa and an infraspinous fossa.
- Depending on the degree of scapular protraction/retraction, the edge of the scapular blade can be seen anywhere from anterior to the vertebral column and close to the tracheo-oesophageal line to posterior to the vertebral column.

▪ Question 4: Axial MRI of the knee

Answer: Semimembranosus

- The semimembranosus muscle originates from a thick tendon from the ischial tuberosity.
- This proximal tendon forms an aponeurotic covering on the anterior aspect of the muscle, which unites to form a distal tendon that inserts into the posterior aspect of the medial condyle of the tibia.
- Baker cysts (popliteal cysts) are fluid-filled bursae lined by synovium that are found between the semimembranosus and medial head of the gastrocnemius muscle tendons.

■ Question 5: Axial CT of the abdomen

Answer: Right renal artery

- In this image, you can see two vessels between the right kidney and the great vessels. To determine whether the vessel is the renal vein or artery, look at the calibre of the vessels and their position.
- The renal artery is normally of a smaller diameter than the renal vein. The artery is also usually posterior to the vein.
- The right renal artery passes posterior to the inferior vena cava—an important landmark for ultrasound.

■ Question 6: Sagittal T1-weighted MRI of the brain

Answer: Fourth ventricle

- The fourth ventricle is a triangular-shaped structure on the sagittal view.
- It is bordered by the pons and medulla anteriorly, the superior cerebellar peduncles superiorly, and the inferior cerebellar peduncles inferiorly.

■ Question 7: Plain radiograph of the sternum

Answer: Sternum

- The sternum is a tie-shaped bone that forms the midportion of the anterior thoracic cage.
- It articulates with the clavicles and the costal cartilages of the first seven ribs.
- It has a manubrium, body, and xiphoid process.
- Oblique views such as this are necessary to project the sternum away from the heart. Lateral views are also sometimes used.

■ Question 8: Coronal MRI of the pelvis

Answer: Right gracilis muscle

- The long and thin gracilis muscle arises from the ischiopubic ramus and inserts via the conjoint tendon known as the pes anserinus onto the anteromedial aspect of the proximal tibia.

Question 9: Axial CT of the abdomen

Answer: Left external oblique muscle

- The external oblique muscle is the outermost abdominal muscle. Its fibres run obliquely from supero-lateral to inferomedial, crossing the fibres of the internal oblique muscle at approximately 90°.
- It forms a large aponeurosis with the other lateral abdominal muscles, which becomes the rectus sheath as it envelopes the rectus abdominis muscle.
- The order of the lateral abdominal muscles from superficial to deep layer is: external oblique, internal oblique, transversus abdominis.

Question 10: Axial T2-weighted MRI of the brain

Answer: Medulla oblongata

- On axial images, it can be difficult to determine the level of the brainstem on a single slice. The key is to look at the shape of the section of brainstem and also the surrounding anatomy.
- The medulla is the most inferior portion of the brainstem. Some of the surrounding structures to take note of are the maxillary antra and the mandibular condyles, which indicate the inferior position in the skull.
- The medulla connects to the pons (superiorly) and to the spinal cord (inferiorly) at the level of the foramen magnum.
- It lies anterior to the fourth ventricle.
- It has connections to the cerebellum via the inferior cerebellar peduncles (pictured).
- Its ventral surface is made up of the pyramids (anteromedially) and the olives (posterolaterally).

Question 11: Coronal CT of the chest

Answer: Right subclavian artery

- The right subclavian artery, as its name suggests, passes underneath the clavicle, a part of which can be seen on this image.
- It ascends superolaterally from its origin at the brachiocephalic artery to pass through the anterior part of the scalene triangle between scalenus medius and scalenus anterior and crosses the first rib. Distal to this point, it becomes the right axillary artery.

Question 12: Axial MRI of the pelvis

Answer: Left rectus femoris

- The large rectus femoris muscle originates from the anterior inferior iliac spine and iliac portion of the acetabulum.
- It is part of the quadriceps femoris—the other muscles being vastus lateralis, vastus medialis, and vastus intermedius.
- The rectus femoris muscle is placed centrally and is the most superficial of the quadriceps muscles.
- The quadriceps muscles insert into the tibial tuberosity via the common patellar tendon.

■ Question 13: US of the abdomen

Answer: Gallbladder

- Ultrasound is the principal investigation for assessment of the gallbladder.
- The gallbladder is located on the inferior surface of the liver. The normal wall thickness of a full gall-bladder is < 3 mm.
- The gallbladder consists of the neck, body, and fundus.
- The gallbladder lumen should contain anechoic fluid.
- It forms one point of the Cantlie line, which divides the left and right lobe of the liver.

■ Question 14: Axial CT of the neck

Answer: Left vertebral artery

- The left vertebral artery is the first branch of the subclavian artery and supplies the brainstem, cerebellum, and spinal cord.
- It enters the foramen transversarium of C6 and ascends through the foramina of the more superior vertebrae to enter the skull.
- The two vertebral arteries merge to form the basilar artery in the pre-pontine cistern.
- The left vertebral artery is larger than the right in 40% of patients, and the arteries are equal in size in 40% of patients.

■ Question 15: Coronal MRI of the brain

Answer: Right internal carotid artery

- The internal carotid artery lies lateral to the optic chiasm and superior to the sphenoid sinuses.
- It is divided into four segments:
  - **Cervical:** arises posterolaterally from the bifurcation of the common carotid artery at the level of C4 and has no branches
  - **Petrous:** through the foramen lacerum
  - **Cavernous:** through the cavernous sinus
  - **Supraclinoid**

▪ Question 16: Axial MRI of the right knee

Answer: Tendon of the right sartorius muscle

- Sartorius is the longest muscle in the human body. It is a superficial thigh muscle that originates from the anterior superior iliac spine and inserts via a conjoint tendon known as the pes anserinus onto the anteromedial aspect of the proximal tibia.
- The pes anserinus ('goose's foot') is a conjoint tendon and composed of tendons from three muscles (from anterior to posterior): sartorius, gracilis, and semitendinosus. There are various mnemonics for this arrangement, such as 'Say Grace before Tea'.
- Note that all three contributory tendons of the pes anserinus pass behind the medial femoral condyle.

▪ Question 17: US of the abdomen

Answer: Head of pancreas

- The head of the pancreas lies to the right of the neck, which is defined by the confluence of the superior mesenteric vein and splenic vein.
- The common bile duct and pancreatic duct pass through the head of the pancreas, which lies in contact with the descending portion of the duodenum.

▪ Question 18: Sagittal T1-weighted MRI of the brain

Answer: Anterior pituitary gland

- The pituitary gland is located in the sella turcica (Latin for 'Turkish saddle'), inferior to the optic chiasm.
- It is connected to the hypothalamus via the infundibulum (stalk).
- It demonstrates strong contrast enhancement because it is not contained within the blood–brain barrier.
- The posterior pituitary gland is bright on a T1-weighted (unenhanced) scan.

▪ Question 19: Coronal CT of the chest

Answer: Right atrium

- You can see the inferior vena cava at the inferior aspect of this cardiac chamber, which tells you that this is the right atrium as opposed to the right ventricle.
- The right atrium sits more posteriorly than the right ventricle, which cannot be seen in this image.

Question 20: T1-weighted sagittal MRI of the knee

Answer: Posterior cruciate ligament

- The function of the posterior cruciate ligament (PCL) is to resist hyperflexion of the knee.
- It arises from the posterior aspect of the intercondylar area of the tibia.
- It attaches to the inner surface of the medial femoral condyle.
- The PCL is less affected by the magic angle effect when compared with the anterior cruciate ligament and therefore appears as a solid black band on MRI.

Question 21: Mammogram

Answer: Glandular breast tissue

- The glandular tissue is covered anteriorly by subcutaneous fat. Posteriorly, there is retroglandular fat and then the pectoralis major muscle.
- The glandular tissue is comprised of 15 to 20 lobes that are formed of multiple lobules, which drain many acini.
- The blood supply to the breast comes from branches of the internal mammary and the lateral thoracic artery (a branch of the axillary artery).

Question 22: Barium meal

Answer: Gastric antrum

- The stomach has two curvatures: the lesser and greater.
- The oesophagus joins the stomach at the gastro-oesophageal junction—also known as the cardia—at the upper aspect of the lesser curvature.
- The fundus is the most superior part of the stomach, followed by the body and then the antrum. The pylorus is a continuation of the antrum, which opens into the duodenum.

Question 23: Coronal MRI of the brain (FLAIR sequence)

Answer: Right lacrimal gland

- The lacrimal gland is an almond-shaped gland that lies in the lacrimal fossa of the frontal bone, in the superolateral aspect of each orbit.
- It secretes the aqueous layer of the tear film.

■ Question 24: Angiogram of the right lower limb

Answer: Right anterior tibial artery

- There are three main branches of the popliteal artery: the anterior tibial artery arises first, followed by the tibioperoneal trunk, which gives rise to the posterior tibial and peroneal arteries.
- These three main branches correlate to their respective fascial compartments of the leg.

■ Question 25: T2-weighted sagittal MRI of the head

Answer: Sphenoid sinus

- At first glance, this structure may seem difficult to identify, but it is easy to work out.
- The image shows a midline sagittal slice with the arrow pointing to a very low signal intensity structure similar to that outside the patient—that is, air.
- The only midline air-filled structures are the frontal (also pictured) and sphenoid sinuses. The ethmoid sinuses are paramidline and consist of many small air cells.

■ Question 26: Axial CT of the chest

Answer: Right supraspinatus muscle

- The supraspinatus is a small muscle that runs obliquely from the supraspinous fossa to insert at the greater tuberosity of the humerus.
- It is separated from the infraspinatus muscle by the spine of the scapula. On axial CT images, it is medial to the spine of the scapula and dorsal to the subscapularis muscle.

■ Question 27: Ultrasound of the neck

Answer: Left common carotid artery

- This image shows the left side of the neck. Initially, the appearances are confusing, but if you take time to examine the structures, you will recognise the tracheal ring on the left of the image, the hyperreflective left lobe of the thyroid, and the anechoic vessels to the right of the image.
- The common carotid artery is more rounded and smaller in diameter compared with the internal jugular vein.

Question 28: Chest radiograph

Answer: Azygos fissure

- The appearance of the azygos fissure is more subtle on a plain radiograph compared with a CT scan.
- The location and tear-drop shape with a radio-opaque line emerging from its superior aspect is characteristic.
- The azygos fissure comprises four layers of pleura: two parietal and two visceral.

Question 29: Axial MRI arthrogram of the right hip

Answer: Gluteus maximus

- The gluteus maximus muscle is a largely superficial muscle that originates from a large area of the posterior pelvis (gluteal surface of the iliac bone, sacrum and coccyx, the sacrotuberous ligament, and the lumbar fascia).
- It inserts into the iliotibial band of the fascia lata, as well as a deeper site at the gluteus tuberosity of the femur.

Question 30: Axial T2-weighted MRI of the brain

Answer: Anterior limb of the right internal capsule

- This is a white matter tract that separates the caudate (medially) from the lentiform nucleus (laterally).
- It returns a lower signal on T2-weighted imaging relative to the lentiform nucleus.

Question 31: Axial contrast-enhanced CT of the chest

Answer: Circumflex artery

- The circumflex artery is the other main branch of the left coronary artery.
- It runs in the posterior atrioventricular groove to the posterior surface of the heart where it anastomoses with the right coronary artery.
- It supplies blood to the left atrium and left ventricle.

Question 32: Mesenteric angiogram

Answer: Splenic artery

- The splenic artery is one of the three branches of the coeliac trunk. The left gastric artery and common hepatic artery are the others.
- Usually it is a much more tortuous artery than seen in this image.
- You can be certain that it is the splenic artery and not the left renal artery because of the outline of the organ and the overlying left dome of the diaphragm. The right renal pelvis can also be seen to the bottom right of the picture.

Question 33: Axial CT of the neck

Answer: Body of the hyoid bone

- The hyoid bone can be recognised as a horseshoe-shaped structure that lies between the mandible and the thyroid cartilage.
- It has a central body and greater cornua or horns on either side.
- The lesser cornua of the hyoid arise from the junction of the body and greater cornua more superiorly.

Question 34: Coronal MRI of the pelvis

Answer: Left obturator externus

- The obturator externus muscle originates from the lateral aspect of the obturator foramen and obturator membrane.
- It passes posterolaterally before inserting into the trochanteric fossa of the greater trochanter of the femur.
- On this image, obturator internus is the muscle superior to it.

Question 35: Axial contrast-enhanced CT of the chest

Answer: Coronary sinus

- The aorta and left ventricle are full of contrast medium, whereas the arrowed structure is not; therefore, it must contain venous blood. It is draining into the right atrium, which means it is the coronary sinus.
- The coronary sinus drains into the posterior wall of the right atrium.
- Its tributaries include the great, middle, and small cardiac veins and the left posterior ventricular vein.
- The anterior cardiac veins drain directly into the anterior wall of the right atrium.

■ Question 36: PA chest radiograph

Answer: Right paratracheal stripe

- The right paratracheal stripe is the interface between the right upper lobe and the right lateral tracheal border.
- The maximum width is 5 mm. It should be uniform and not nodular.
- The left lateral wall is not usually visible on chest X-ray.

■ Question 37: Axial T2-weighted MRI of the brain

Answer: Right putamen

- The putamen lies lateral to the anterior limb of the internal capsule and anterolateral to the globus pallidus.
- Putamen + caudate nucleus = striatum
- Putamen + globus pallidus = lentiform nucleus

■ Question 38: MRI of the neck

Answer: Epiglottis

- The epiglottis marks the entrance of the larynx.
- In this image, the glossoepiglottic mucosal fold, which can be seen emerging from the midportion of the epiglottis, connects the epiglottis to the tongue and forms the valleculae on either side.
- The space posterior to the epiglottis is the laryngopharynx/hypopharynx.

■ Question 39: Axial contrast-enhanced CT of the chest

Answer: Left inferior pulmonary vein

- The pulmonary veins drain oxygenated blood from the lungs into the left atrium.
- There are usually four pulmonary veins: two superior and two inferior; however, this can vary. There may be five or six.
- The inferior pulmonary veins run a horizontal course into the left atrium compared with the more oblique course of the superior pulmonary veins.

■ Question 40: Lateral radiograph of the cervical spine

Answer: Dens/odontoid process/odontoid peg

- The second cervical vertebra (axis/C2) is characterised by the dens—a bony projection that arises perpendicularly from the vertebral body.
- Lying immediately anterior to the dens is the anterior arch of the first cervical vertebra (atlas/C1).
- There is a pivot articulation between the dens and the ring formed anteriorly by the anterior arch, and posteriorly by the transverse ligament of C1. This articulation is part of the atlantoaxial joint that allows C1 to rotate on C2.

▪ Question 41: Axial CT of the chest

Answer: Right lower lobe

- The lower lobe is separated from the upper and middle lobes by the oblique fissure.
- It is divided into five segments: apical, anterior basal, lateral basal, posterior basal, and medial basal segments.

▪ Question 42: MR angiogram of the circle of Willis (MIP image)

Answer: Left middle cerebral artery

- The middle cerebral artery (MCA) is the largest branch of the internal carotid artery.
- It does not actually form one of the sides of the pentagon that is the circle of Willis.
- Instead, it branches from the internal carotid artery and travels laterally into the insula toward the cortex where it terminates.
- The MCA and its branches supply the basal ganglia, the anterior part of the internal capsule, the lateral cerebral cortex, the anterior temporal lobe, and the insular cortex.
- The segment from the origin to the bifurcation/trifurcation is referred to as the M1 segment (as shown in the image).

▪ Question 43: CT of the neck in bone window

Answer: Larynx

- The larynx is part of the respiratory tract and lies between the laryngopharynx/hypopharynx and the trachea at the level of C3 to C6.
- It is composed of an articulated cartilaginous skeleton (thyroid, cricoid, and arytenoid cartilages) and various fibroelastic membranes and muscles.
- All three cartilages of the larynx can be seen in the image.
- The larynx is divided into three parts: the supraglottic level, the glottic level, and the infraglottic level.
- The image shows the glottic level, which can be recognised by the triangular shape of the larynx formed by the open vocal cords on either side.

▪ Question 44: Transvaginal US of the uterus in the sagittal plane

Answer: Myometrium

- The uterus is a muscular extraperitoneal organ that lies between the bladder and the rectum.
- The myometrium can be differentiated from the endometrium because it is much thicker and relatively hyporeflective.
- On an ultrasound, the myometrium has homogeneous reflectivity, and fine echo-poor vessels can sometimes be seen within it.

■ Question 45: Sagittal MRI of the shoulder

Answer: Subscapularis muscle

- Subscapularis is a rotator cuff muscle.
- It has a fanlike formation.
- It originates from the subscapular fossa of the scapula and is traditionally said to insert into the lesser tuberosity of the humerus only. However, part of its tendon actually passes farther over the bicipital groove to insert into the greater tuberosity, thereby holding the biceps brachii tendon in place.

■ Question 46: Mammogram

Answer: Pectoralis major muscle

- The pectoral muscles form the anterolateral chest wall.
- Pectoralis major is the larger, more anterior of the two muscles—the other being pectoralis minor.
- Two thirds of the breast rests on the pectoralis major. The other third rests on serratus anterior, more laterally.

■ Question 47: Sagittal MRI of the knee

Answer: Quadriceps tendon

- The four quadriceps muscles—rectus femoris, vastus lateralis, vastus intermedius, and vastus medialis—combine together to form a conjoined tendon, the quadriceps tendon.
- The quadriceps tendon is often described as inserting onto the superior pole of the patella. In actuality, the patella is a sesamoid bone, which sits within the quadriceps tendon. The patellar tendon is a continuation of the quadriceps tendon.

■ Question 48: PA chest radiograph

Answer: Carina

- The carina is where the trachea divides into the right and left main bronchus.
- It lies at the level of T5 and is at the level of the sternal angle.
- The carinal angle measures approximately 65°. Widening of the carinal angle above 65° is a mark of left atrial enlargement or a subcarinal mass.

■ Question 49: Axial T2-weighted MRI of the brain

Answer: Genu of corpus callosum

- The genu is the anterior pole of the corpus callosum.
- *Genu* is Latin for 'knee'. Notice its shape when viewed in the sagittal plane.

■ Question 50: Sagittal T2-weighted MRI of the neck

Answer: Oropharynx

- The oropharynx is the part of the pharynx that lies between the nasopharynx (superior) and laryngopharynx (inferior).
- It extends from the free edge of the soft palate to the superior border of the epiglottis.
- The posterior third of the tongue forms the anterior wall of the oropharynx.
- Note the fracture-dislocation at C4/5.

■ Question 51: Aortic angiogram

Answer: Superior rectal artery

- The superior rectal artery is the terminal branch of the inferior mesenteric artery (IMA).
- Branches and distribution of the IMA are listed below.

From left to right:

Left colic artery	Mid-transverse and descending colon
Sigmoid arteries	Descending and sigmoid colon
Superior rectal artery	Proximal rectum

- The terminal branches of the ileocolic, right colic, and middle colic (all from the superior mesenteric artery) and the left colic and sigmoid arteries (IMA) anastomose to form the marginal artery of Drummond.

■ Question 52: Sagittal MRI of the shoulder

Answer: Supraspinatus muscle

- The supraspinatus muscle is one of the four rotator cuff muscles of the shoulder.
- The supraspinatus originates from the supraspinous fossa. Its tendon passes beneath the acromion and inserts into the greater tuberosity of the humerus.
- Due to its superficial location, it is well visualised on US as well as CT and MRI.
- It can be imaged in various axes on MRI. Look out for its location relative to the acromion on the coronal view and its position relative to the triangular configuration of the spine of the scapula/clavicle and coracoid process on the sagittal view.
- A dedicated coronal oblique view of the shoulder may be performed in the axis of the supraspinatus muscle.

■ Question 53: Axial CT of the chest

Answer: Left main bronchus

- The left main bronchus arises from the trachea at the carina.
- It lies at about 40° to the median plane.
- It is approximately 5 cm long and 1.2 cm in diameter—considerably longer than the right main bronchus.

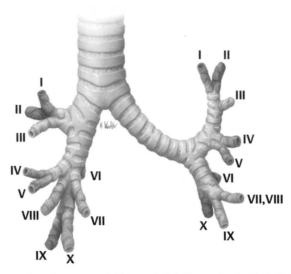

From Atlas of Anatomy, © Thieme 2008, illustration by Karl Wesker.

Segmental architecture of the lungs				
Each segment is supplied by a segmental bronchus of the same name (e.g., the apical segmental bronchus supplies the apical segment).				
	Right lung		**Left lung**	
		Superior lobe		
I	Apical segment	Apicoposterior segment		I
II	Posterior segment			II
III		Anterior segment		III
	Middle lobe		**Lingula**	
IV	Lateral segment	Superior lingular segment		IV
V	Medial segment	Inferior lingular segment		V
		Inferior lobe		
VI		Superior segment		VI
VII		Medial basal segment		VII
VIII		Anterior basal segment		VIII
IX		Lateral basal segment		IX
X		Posterior basal segment		X

■ Question 54: Sagittal T1-weighted MRI of the brain

Answer: Corpus callosum

- The corpus callosum is a midline C-shaped structure that is composed of a flat bundle of nerve fibres.

■ Question 55: MRI arthrogram of the right shoulder

Answer: Right shoulder joint capsule

- The glenohumeral joint capsule is composed of a soft tissue layer lined by synovial membrane.
- The capsule is loose, which permits an increased range of movement.
- The cranial and caudal aspects of the capsule are relatively thick.
- The capsule is reinforced cranially by the coracohumeral ligament, and anteriorly by the glenohumeral ligaments.

■ Question 56: Mesenteric angiogram

Answer: Superior mesenteric artery

- The superior mesenteric artery (SMA) is the second branch of the aorta and usually originates immediately beneath the coeliac trunk (also pictured).
- The SMA runs an anteroinferior course.
- The renal arteries are seen inferiorly to the SMA.
- The table here lists the aortic branches and their usual levels of origin.

Artery	Level of origin
Coeliac trunk	T12
Superior mesenteric artery	L1
Renal arteries	L1/2
Inferior mesenteric artery	L3

- See question 37 in Chapter 3 for branches of the SMA.

■ Question 57: US of the male pelvis

Answer: Prostate gland

- The prostate gland can be recognised as a rounded, midline structure with homogeneous reflectivity, inferior to the urinary bladder, which is the large anechoic structure in the image.
- The gland is composed of four zones: the peripheral, central, and transition zone and the anterior fibromuscular stroma. These cannot be resolved on a transabdominal US.
- The urethra runs through the centre of the prostate gland.

■ Question 58: Orthopantomogram

Answer: Left mandibular condyle

- The mandibular condyle articulates with the mandibular fossa of the temporal bone to make the temporomandibular joint.
- Do not confuse them with the coronoid processes, which are seen medial to the mandibular condyles on the orthopantomogram.

Question 59: Plain radiograph of the right elbow

Answer: Right radial tuberosity

- The proximal diaphysis of the radius is marked on its medial aspect by the radial tuberosity, which is situated just beneath the neck and serves as the insertion site of the biceps brachii muscle.

Question 60: Axial CT of the chest

Answer: Pericardium

- The pericardium is a fibrous bag consisting of a parietal pericardium and a visceral pericardium (epicardium) that surrounds the heart.
- On a CT, the normal pericardium can be seen as a thin sheet of soft tissue density surrounding the heart.

Question 61: Axial T2-weighted MRI of the brain

Answer: Cisterna magna

- The cisterna magna is a cerebrospinal fluid–filled arachnoid space in the posterior fossa.
- It is situated between the cerebellar hemispheres and posterior to the inferior aspect of the medulla.
- It is connected to the fourth ventricle via the foramina of Luschka and Magendie.

Question 62: Axial T1-weighted MRI of the neck

Answer: Right external jugular vein

- At the level of the mandible, the posterior branch of the retromandibular vein and the posterior auricular vein join to form the external jugular vein.
- It is superficial to the sternocleidomastoid muscle.
- It terminates above the midpoint of the clavicle where it joins the subclavian vein.
- The external jugular vein drains the scalp and face.

Question 63: Plain radiograph of the left upper limb

Answer: Greater tuberosity of the left humerus

- The anterolateral convex surface of the humerus is divided by the bicipital groove into two tuberosities: the larger laterally situated greater tuberosity and the smaller medially situated lesser tuberosity.
- Three of the four rotator cuff muscles insert into the greater tuberosity: supraspinatus, infraspinatus, and teres minor (a mnemonic is SIT). The fourth rotator cuff muscle, subscapularis, inserts into the lesser tuberosity.

Question 64: Axial T1-weighted MRI of the neck

Answer: Right parotid gland

- The parotid gland returns a high signal on T1-weighted MRI because of its high fat content.
- It lies posterior to the angle of the mandible and has deep and superficial portions.
- The gland is divided into deep and superficial lobes by the branches of the facial nerve, which run through the gland.
- The external carotid artery and posterior facial vein also run through the parotid gland.

Question 65: Axial CT of the chest

Answer: Right internal thoracic artery (internal mammary artery)

- The right internal thoracic artery is a small calibre artery arising from the right subclavian artery and supplying the right breast and chest wall.
- It runs approximately 1 cm lateral and parallel to the sternum.
- The artery usually runs lateral to the vein up to T4; the vein then crosses over beyond T4. However, there are common anatomical variants.
- The arterial phase appearance of the other vascular structures such as the aortic arch should help differentiate the artery from the vein.
- The internal thoracic vessels (and their accompanying lymph nodes) are important to recognise as they are a bleeding hazard in anterior mediastinal percutaneous biopsies.

Question 66: Axial CT of the brain

Answer: Pineal gland

- The pineal gland is a small (< 1 cm) endocrine gland that is shaped like a pine cone, hence its name.
- It is found in the midline, posterior to the third ventricle, and between the left and right thalami.
- It is calcified in approximately 50% of the population by the age of 20 (as shown in the image).

Question 67: Transvaginal US of the uterus

Answer: Uterine fundus

- The uterus is divided into the fundus (the rounded roof of the uterus), the body (the main bulk of the organ), and the cervix.
- To the untrained eye, it may be difficult to decide which end is the fundus and which end is the cervix. The fundus is the widest part of the uterus.
- It would be useful to become familiar with some of the normal variants in uterine structure—for example, a unicornuate and a bicornuate uterus.
- The cursors measure the endometrial thickness.

Question 68: Plain radiograph of the left foot

Answer: Left os trigonum

- This is a secondary bony ossicle posterior to the talus, which appears between 7 and 12 years of age. It usually fuses with the talus. Those that do not fuse are known as os trigonum.

Question 69: MR venogram (MIP image)

Answer: Transverse sinus

- The left and right transverse sinuses emerge from the confluence of the sinuses.
- The right is usually a continuation of the superior sagittal sinus, whereas the left is usually continuous with the straight sinus.
- It is not possible to determine whether this is the left or the right transverse sinus in the image.
- Where the sinus takes a downward turn in the mastoid bone is referred to as the sigmoid sinus.
- Once the sigmoid sinus has passed through the jugular foramen, it becomes the internal jugular vein.

Question 70: MRA of the circle of Willis (MIP image)

Answer: Right posterior cerebral artery

- The posterior cerebral arteries (PCAs) are terminal branches of the basilar artery.
- The PCAs complete the circle of Willis by joining the internal carotid arteries via the posterior communicating arteries.
- The PCA supplies the inferior occipital and temporal lobes.

Question 71: Plain film of the wrist

Answer: Lunate bone

- The lunate bone is one of the eight carpal bones.
- It is situated between the scaphoid and triquetral bones.
- The scapholunate joint should be < 3 mm. If this space is widened, it is suggestive of scapholunate dislocation.

▪ Question 72: Axial CT of the chest

Answer: Horizontal fissure

- The horizontal fissure separates the right upper lobe from the middle lobe and usually extends from the level of the 6th rib.
- It courses from the right hilum to the right lateral anterior chest wall and can sometimes be seen on PA and lateral chest radiographs, particularly when it contains pleural fluid.
- It is important to recognise the normal anatomical position of the horizontal fissure because it moves upward in apical fibrosis of the right upper lobe and moves downward in atelectasis of the lower lobe.

▪ Question 73: Sagittal T2-weighted MRI of the brain

Answer: Quadrigeminal (tectal) plate

- The quadrigeminal plate is the dorsal portion of the midbrain.
- It is made up of the paired superior and inferior colliculi. It is responsible for visual and auditory reflexes.
- The quadrigeminal plate is located within the quadrigeminal cistern.

▪ Question 74: MR angiogram with MIP image of the circle of Willis

Answer: Basilar artery

- It is vital to memorise the components that form the circle of Willis because it is a common examination question.
- The basilar artery is an unpaired vessel that is formed by the union of the two vertebral arteries.
- It lies close to the midline in most people but can deviate to one side away from the dominant vertebral artery.
- It terminates by dividing into the left and right posterior cerebral arteries.

▪ Question 75: Oblique radiograph of the foot

Answer: Right navicular bone

- Navicular, as its name suggests, is a boat-shaped tarsal bone found on the medial aspect of the foot.
- It articulates proximally with the talus, distally with the cuneiform bones, and laterally with the cuboid bone.
- An accessory navicular bone is a common finding seen in approximately 10% of the population.

■ Question 76: Axial CT of the brain

Answer: Right interventricular foramen of Monro

- The foramen of Monro is a paired structure that connects the left and right lateral ventricles to the third ventricle.
- It forms the anterior border of the third ventricle.

■ Question 77: Sagittal T2-weighted MRI of the brain

Answer: Cerebellar tonsil

- The cerebellar tonsil is the most inferior lobule of the cerebellar hemisphere.
- It lies posterior to the medulla.
- Its inferior tip lies above or at the level of the foramen magnum.

■ Question 78: Barium swallow

Answer: Aortic arch

- Three structures indent the left side of the oesophagus.
- The most superior structure as shown in the image is the aortic arch.
- The next indentation down is caused by the left main bronchus—this concavity is usually more shallow.
- The next indentation is more subtle and is caused by the left atrium.

■ Question 79: MR venogram

Answer: Straight sinus

- The straight sinus is situated at the junction of the falx cerebri and the tentorium cerebelli.
- It receives blood from the inferior sagittal sinus and the great cerebral vein of Galen.
- In this example, the straight sinus is draining into the left transverse sinus, but it can also drain into the confluence of the sinuses or the right transverse sinus.

■ Question 80: Coronal CT of the abdomen (MIP image)

Answer: Two accessory renal arteries

- In the image, there are three renal arteries supplying the right kidney.
- Accessory renal arteries are the most common renal vascular variants, seen in approximately one third of the population.
- These accessory arteries take origin from the abdominal aorta, but they can also arise from the coeliac axis, mesenteric, lumbar, middle colic, or middle sacral artery.

■ Question 81: AP radiograph of the left foot

Answer: Left fifth metatarsal

- As with the other four metatarsal, the fifth metatarsal can be divided into base, shaft, and head.
- Peroneus brevis and peroneus tertius muscle tendons insert into the base.

■ Question 82: Coronal MRI of the brain

Answer: Aqueduct of Sylvius (cerebral aqueduct)

- The aqueduct of Sylvius is a thin, midline tube that connects the third ventricle to the fourth ventricle.
- It is located in the midbrain between the pons (anterior) and the cerebellum (posterior).
- It is filled with cerebrospinal fluid.

■ Question 83: Coronal CT of the chest

Answer: Bronchus suis (pig's bronchus)

- In this patient, the right upper lobe bronchus takes origin from the trachea rather than from the right main bronchus.
- This variant has a frequency of approximately 0.2% and occurs much more frequently on the right.
- It is more common in males and can be associated with other congenital abnormalities.

■ Question 84: Coronal FLAIR MRI of the brain

Answer: Left cerebellar hemisphere

- The cerebellum is an infratentorial structure in the posterior fossa.
- It is separated by the median cerebellar vermis into the right and left cerebellar hemispheres.
- The cerebellar hemispheres are separated into lobules by fissures (folia).
- The cerebellum is connected to the brainstem via three cerebellar peduncles:
  - Superior peduncle connects to the midbrain
  - Middle peduncle connects to the pons
  - Inferior peduncle connects to the base of the pons

Question 85: AP radiograph of the right hand

Answer: Right scapholunate joint

- There are eight carpal bones in each hand arranged in two rows. The scaphoid, lunate, triquetral, and pisiform bones in the proximal row. The trapezium, trapezoid, capitate, and hamate in the distal row.
- The intercarpal joints can be divided into joints within the proximal row, distal row, and those between the two rows.
- The wrist joint allows complex patterns of movement. Stability of the wrist joint is achieved by the interlocking shape of each carpal bone and a strong ligamentous apparatus.
- The bones in each row effectively function as a single articular body.
- Alternatively, the carpus is divisible into three columns: radial scaphoid column (scaphoid-trapezium-trapezoid), lunate (lunate-capitate), and ulnar triquetral column (triquetrum-hamate). This format is useful when examining the carpus on the lateral view. You should be able to identify the scaphoid, lunate, and capitate on a lateral plain radiograph.

Question 86: Axial CT of the neck

Answer: Left transverse process of atlas (C1)

- The atlas is unique in its structure and readily identifiable on a single axial image.
- The anterior and posterior tubercles typical of C3-C7 vertebrae are fused in the atlas to form a relatively large process that projects laterally and inferiorly from the lateral mass.
- Each transverse process contains the foramen transversarium, which transmits the vertebral artery, vertebral vein, and nerves.

Question 87: Sagittal T2-weighted MRI of the brain

Answer: Cingulate gyrus

- The cingulate gyrus is a midline curved structure that lies inferior to the frontal lobes and superior to the corpus callosum.
- It is separated from the corpus callosum by the cingulate sulcus.
- The cingulate gyrus forms part of the limbic system.

Question 88: Axial MRI of the neck

Answer: Right vallecula

- Just visible on the image is the central glossoepiglottic fold, which passes from the anterior surface of the epiglottis to the base of the tongue.
- This forms a pair of recesses between the tongue and the epiglottis called the valleculae.
- The valleculae form a temporary trap for saliva to prevent initiation of the swallowing reflex.

■ Question 89: Sagittal MRI of the cervicothoracic spine

Answer: T5 vertebral body

- You can determine the number of the vertebrae by counting down from the odontoid process of C2.
- There are 24 articulating vertebrae within the vertebral column: 7 cervical, 12 thoracic, and 5 lumbar. There are five sacral and four coccygeal bones that are not separated by intervertebral discs and are fused.

■ Question 90: Occipitomental radiograph of the face

Answer: Right frontal sinus

- The frontal sinuses are mucosa-lined airspaces in the frontal bone.
- They are located above the orbits and form part of the paranasal sinuses.
- They vary in shape and are usually paired.

■ Question 91: Sagittal T1-weighted MRI of the brain

Answer: Nasopharynx

- The nasopharynx is the most superior portion of the pharynx.
- It extends from the skull base to the soft palate and is connected to the nasal cavities.
- It lies anterior to the pharyngeal tonsils (most prominent in childhood).

■ Question 92: AP radiograph of left hand

Answer: Epiphysis of the proximal phalanx of the left little finger

- The image is a radiograph of a child's hand. It is important to know the names of the different parts of the bones including epiphysis, metaphysis, diaphysis, and the physis.
- With this type of image, you should aim to provide as much information as possible, similar to that given in this answer.

■ Question 93: Axial T2-weighted MRI of the brain

Answer: Prepontine cistern

- The prepontine cistern is a cerebrospinal fluid–filled space that lies anterior to the pons.
- It contains the basilar artery and two of its paired branches: the anterior inferior cerebellar artery and superior cerebellar arteries.
- The abducens nerve (CN VI) traverses it.

▪ Question 94: MRI of the right wrist

Answer: Right flexor digitorum superficialis tendons

- The palmar aspect of the carpus is concave and covered by the flexor retinaculum forming the carpal tunnel, which contains nine flexor tendons: flexor digitorum superficialis (4), flexor digitorum profundus (4), and flexor pollicis longus (1).
- The flexor digitorum superficialis and profundus muscle tendons pass through a laterally positioned common ulnar sheath, whereas the flexor carpi radialis passes through a medially placed radial sheath.
- The median nerve traverses the carpal tunnel deep to the flexor retinaculum and superficial to the flexor tendons.

▪ Question 95: Axial T2-weighted MRI of the brain

Answer: Pons

- The pons is the mid-portion of the brainstem and connects the midbrain (superiorly) and the medulla (inferiorly).
- It lies posterior to the prepontine cistern and anterior to the fourth ventricle.
- It is located between the two temporal lobes.
- The pons is connected to the cerebellar hemispheres posteriorly via the middle cerebellar peduncles (pictured) and the inferior cerebellar peduncles.

▪ Question 96: Sagittal MRI of the brain

Answer: Medulla

- The medulla is the most inferior portion of the brainstem.
- It connects the pons (superiorly) to the spinal cord (inferiorly at the level of the foramen magnum).
- It lies anterior to the fourth ventricle.
- Its ventral surface is made up of the pyramids (anteromedial) and the olives (posterolaterally).
- Its posterior portion contains the nucleus gracilis (medial) and nucleus cuneatus (lateral).

▪ Question 97: Coronal MRI of the brain

Answer: Right internal capsule

- The internal capsule separates the caudate (medially) and the lentiform nucleus (laterally).
- It returns a lower signal on T2-weighted image relative to the lentiform nucleus.

▪ Question 98: Coronal MR enterography

Answer: Appendix

- The appendix is a blind-ended tubular structure of variable length.
- The normal appendix has a maximal diameter of 6 mm with a maximum wall thickness of 3 mm.
- It can lie in virtually any orientation from the caecum.
- It is supplied by the ileocolic vessels from the superior mesenteric artery. The lymphatic supply follows the artery.

▪ Question 99: Coronal T1-weighted MRI of the brain

Answer: Optic chiasm

- The optic chiasm is located in the suprasellar cistern.
- It lies superior to the pituitary gland and anterior to the pituitary stalk (infundibulum).

▪ Question 100: Coronal CT of the brain

Answer: Third ventricle

- The third ventricle is a slitlike structure in the midline.
- The third ventricle is connected to the fourth ventricle via the aqueduct of Sylvius.
- The borders of the third ventricle are:
  - Anterior: columns of fornix, foramina of Monro, anterior commissure, optic chiasm, optic recess, and lamina terminalis
  - Lateral: thalamus (superiorly) and hypothalamus (inferiorly)
  - Roof: body of fornix (medially), choroid fissure, thalamus, and stria medullaris (laterally)
  - Floor: optic chiasm, infundibulum, tuber cinereum, and mamillary bodies
- Its anatomic recesses include the optic recess, infundibular recess, pineal recess, suprapineal recess, and interthalamic adhesion (massa intermedia).

INDEX

Note: Page numbers followed by *f* indicate figures.